FEMDOM: Serve and be Served

A 2-in-1 Book Bundle About the FLR Lifestyle

Alexandra Morris

TABLE OF CONTENTS

Dominant Women

Submissive Men

Being a Submissive Man In The Modern World

not limited to, —errors, omissions, or inaccuracies.

Introduction

Gender roles are constantly changing and this affects not only sexuality in society but gender roles generally are dictated by the labor needs of any civilization. One of the best ways of illustrating this, perhaps, would be a woman's role in the 1940s and '50s, which changed radically and quickly to accommodate the financial and resource requirements of the economy. When men were called to arms to fight in World War II - indeed, in any war - it was women who had to fill in the gaps in the labor market back home, which could necessitate them working in factories and assembling bombs and weapons, for instance.

In the 1950s, after men had returned from the war and had gone back into the labor market, women became surplus to requirements within the labor force and were encouraged instead to stay at home and raise their families. This was reinforced by governments. Even academic research, such as Bowlby's Attachment Theory, seemed to aim at convincing women that their place was in the home looking after the children so that children could form strong attachments to their primary career; their mother of course. This threw the onus of being the breadwinner heavily back onto the male who became the dominant member in the household and who could expect his house to be cleaned, his children to be cared for and a hot meal waiting for him and served up by a wife who had done her best to look pretty for his return. Women were pushed out of the labor force and told to know their place.

This shift in roles can be clearly observed and is well documented in advertising campaigns showing the woman having clearly defined menial tasks and the man adopting the dominant role and leaving the home to do important work. Advertising on the new-fangled television and in magazines demonstrated how deliriously happy women were to have vacuum cleaners and washing machines and soap powders that removed all stains. Even fashion reflected a nipped in waist and dirndl skirts emphasized those lovely child bearing hips and the feminine form of a woman who would appeal to the men she lived to serve.

This quite clearly pervaded into the sexual arena. In the United Kingdom, for instance, there was a commonly used phrase, "Lie back and think of England," intimating that only the man took pleasure from sex and a woman was just doing 'her duty' and wanted to get the actual act over with as soon as possible. Because so many lives had been lost in the war, and men had been absent for long periods, the 1950s produced the generation who later were to become known as the *baby boomers* that enjoyed advantages that had been denied to their predecessors. As more domestic appliances became available, life for women became easier and so men expected them to be looking attractive and for them to be sexually available on demand.

There cannot be anything new under the sun in a sexual

sense. Everything is cyclical and even pedophilia, although largely prohibited and regarded as taboo worldwide now, has at times throughout history been acceptable almost across the globe. Indeed, it is still part of normal society currently in certain parts of the third world and this is precipitated by that society's economic needs. There are huge expanses of women who are never exposed to any formal education and their role is still to look after the menial side of family life.

Women have been the submissive part of a couple for centuries and in an effort to prove a woman's purity practices can be extremely brutal and barbaric. Currently there is no thought or effort put into providing an education for huge swathes of women in third world countries. Their lives are simple and any opportunity to break free from that lifestyle is severely limited. In thirty countries in Africa, Asia and the Middle East, UNICEF estimated that in 2016 there were 200 million women who had been subjected to female genital mutilation (FMG). This is the horrific practice of removing the external parts of female genitalia with a blade and normally occurs within a few days after birth and often before the child is five years old. It occurs mainly in countries, which are Muslim and is performed for cultural, sexual and modesty and purity reasons. The clitoris is often cut away denying sexual gratification for the woman and the vagina is sewn up, leaving a small hole for urination and menstruation. When the man has sex with the girl for the first time he forces himself into the woman. It is mostly done by women who regard it as a great honor and who believe that their daughters and granddaughters must receive this mutilation to escape social exclusion. Needless to say, this causes many health problems and there are no health benefits. There is now international condemnation of this practice. It is hardly surprising that the pendulum is beginning to swing and that women would want to escape from these harsh treatments.

In the 1960s, with the advent of the contraceptive pill for women, roles began to change in the Western world at least. Being in control of when, and even if, to have children, freed women up to enter the labor market themselves. Education became a much more viable option and an increasing number of women were able to enter the upper echelons of commerce and industry, albeit at a lesser salary. Indeed, this financial anomaly still exists today and has quite recently been a hot topic of debate in the western world. Women became independent and realized that they did not actually *need* a man to support them because they were quite capable of doing this for themselves. There have been many countries across the world now that has had a female political leader. While the United Kingdom has had two recently, America came close with an almost-ran, Hillary Clinton.

And still, the emasculation of the male population continues. The contraceptive pill helped to mark the 1960s as *The Swinging Sixties* where anything went and the female population could engage in free sex -

sleeping with anyone she wanted but still gaining the title of slag and slut and any other derogatory banter that might be shared in the golf club, where women were often still not allowed (Gentlemen Only, Ladies Forbidden). Women who were already in the workforce were used to sexual harassment and often a little tap on the backside as they passed someone's desk only earned the offender a title of office "letch." At the very worst, he became a joke amongst the women and a bit of a lad amongst the men. Women's emancipation was all a bit of a joke really because women had always been regarded as common property of the male population to be whistled at in the street and touched up near the photocopier. More recently, there has been an absolute uproar in America and the United Kingdom about male sexual harassment, much of it historical and dating back decades. Harvey Weinstein is perhaps the most famous to be named and shamed and even Donald Trump did not escape condemnation for his pussy grabbing antics but remarkably still went onto become the President of America. So it wasn't really all that serious.

While the earth continues to shift beneath our feet, so too does sexuality and it wasn't until 2003 that the legal rights of LGBT people were recognized in America. Indeed, all levels of sexuality seem to be infiltrating into the modern world sexual arena as minority groups demand recognition of their human rights and are encompassed within the whole. Recognizing our individual feelings and inclinations and making sense of them can be equally daunting and leave us with a sense of feeling abnormal and unsure of how to satisfy needs that may largely be viewed as distasteful or just plain kinky by the larger society.

There are so many factors and influences that make an individual what they are. Each of us is unique and because the topic of male submission has not been openly and freely embraced by society – yet - it can be difficult understanding feelings that do not seem to fit into the mold. This book helps to help answer those questions and should help you realize that if it feels right and does not hurt anyone then just do it. After reading this book, I hope you feel set free to be exactly who you are sexually and realize that enacting fantasies can be enormously liberating and hugely enjoyable.

Chapter One – What is Normal?

When we think of being submissive generally we are more likely to think of women, rather than men but as the world constantly changes, so too does sexuality for both genders. Fifty Shades of Grey has addressed through the medium of pop culture what it means to be a female submissive. And even though ardent feminists are probably vehemently in opposition of the portrayal of women being exploited for cheap thrills on the screen, it does address a part of sexuality that really does need more exposure (forgive the pun).

If we try to define 'normal' there are many more than fifty shades of it. Our sexual preferences are, to a degree, biological but they are also governed by every experience, sexual or otherwise, we have been exposed to throughout our lives. We might try hard to fit the expected norm but an internal struggle can start and if left unexplored can fester and cause psychological problems. Discussion and openness of sexual preferences should be welcomed so that the degrees of normalcy can be identified and accepted by a wider society, not denigrated by ignorance and fear: your own or others'.

It can be exceptionally difficult sometimes to determine what governs your sexual inclinations. The reasons behind sexual preferences and practices are complex and you may not even be aware yourself of what has formed them within your psyche. If laws are introduced to protect society, then we should question more minutely the determinants of those laws as an individual and as a society.

For instance, let us ask why homosexuality should be outlawed? Was it perhaps to protect the traditional format of a family to produce children and maintain a cohesive civilization? Tax laws were introduced to promulgate a traditional family, which in turn was expected to lead to a cohesive law-abiding and financially stable society. And historically, we were all so thoroughly indoctrinated to agree that homosexual practice was abhorrent and a sin against mankind. We are now suffering from overpopulation so there seems to be little requirement for homosexuals to be arrested and locked up for their crime and the law is being relaxed. While homophobia is still very much alive and kicking, more people are at least opening up to its place in a modern society and prosecution is lessening.

However, imagine how much damage that maltreatment has already caused. And that has been achieved by keeping the masses under control and angry at the perceived cause of their deprived plight so that the queers amongst us could be regarded as pariahs. On an individual basis a homosexual, or indeed anyone who does not fit the accepted prescription, could be damaged long term and grow old thinking he or she is perverted and weird. How sad is it to realize that so many people have fallen beyond the realms of happiness because they did not accurately fit into shape that the present economic climate demanded?

The point that should be made here is that homosexuals are not hurting anyone and that there is no reason for them to be persecuted. Prejudice on the grounds of sexuality is as baseless as racial prejudice and no coherent and intelligent argument could be used in its favor. More often than not it is not a conscious decision to be who we are sexually. Our preferences grow with us, but we can be made to feel as if we are outside of societal norms and we desist from doing what we really want or hide it and deny it. As educated as we become about any subject, environmental influences can have a huge bearing on what we internalize and how we come to view ourselves. Can it be reasonably accepted that as long as we are not hurting anyone, we should be free to fulfill our sexual desires with any other consulting adult?

Of course, there will always be those who say that anything other than traditional sexual intercourse, without any kind of perverse behavior, between a man and a woman is wrong. By *traditional* let us assume that means one man and one woman using the missionary position. How boring and unappealing would that be? It can be of no surprise that people who always adopt this position have a special night of the week for it and it is never spontaneous. Repression of natural desires is unhealthy, irrelevant and not required in a society where a happy sex life contributes to a healthy mental and emotional state.

And, on the subject of health, being with a submissive male partner, women are much less likely to suffer from male violence. A survey entitled *the National Crime Victimization Survey* conducted in 2006 and included rapes and sexual assaults that were *not* reported to the police said that 232,960 women reported suffered such crimes, which is more than 600 a day. Another disturbing figure is that there are around 120 million women worldwide who have either been raped or forced to participate in some other sexual act. The perpetrators are most often husbands and boyfriends or former partners. Another startling statistic is that 74% of humans trafficked globally are women and children and nearly 75% of these women and children are used for sexual human trafficking. I could go on but I think these statistics very starkly prove a point that women are still being exploited and used as sexual objects by people who no longer regard them as human. Submissive males begin to sound like a very safe and healthy option for everyone concerned, not least of all for society as a whole.

Equally, wanting to participate in the behavior of a submissive male is only a single facet of sexual normalcy. Each individual has multiple predilections towards myriad behaviors, which can easily change and be dependent on a factor as trivial as mood. We should be grateful that we have freedom of choice, which allows us to be who we truly are and embrace it. Being a submissive male does not have to be hardwired and a regular practice or one-dimensional. It may be something you experiment with and decide to adopt at varying levels in different circumstances and times. At first, it might seem unnatural. You may have been fighting against it all your life up until that first brave moment you decide to relax and enjoy yourself. Even during the act, you might hear that voice inside your head telling you that what you are doing is wrong. Or, conversely, you might regret not having tried it before and wasting time and feeling at once that this is an experience that you are going to embrace and accept into your life on a regular basis.

It's unfortunate that many of us suffer from inhibitions that have no sound basis in fact or commonsense, and yet they are instilled into us and stop us from leading a healthy and fulfilling sex life. It's almost as if that thought has been introduced in much the same way as a habit is learned. You are exposed to the concept over and over again, sometimes consciously but mostly it is insidious and you do not even realize how your opinions are being carved out inside your head. But then an inclination that is at odds with your trained and ingrained thoughts and beliefs is introduced and this is where the conflict can start. For you to be reading this book suggests that you might be at this stage.

But remember, habits can be broken. And that is done by practice and by the acquisition of knowledge and the breaking down of solid barriers to your happiness. This book seeks to provide the answers you might have been looking for and most of them will already be within you. It is about exploring who you are and how you got there. But mostly, it's about who you want to be and how to achieve that, specifically being a submissive male, both sexually and generally.

Of course, there are many professional "Dommes" out there who are very good at what they do and you may choose to experiment with one or more of them. Or you may want to do it within the boundaries of a close relationship where adopting the role of a sexually submissive male adds new and layered dimensions to explore and enjoy, a role that you may like to flip at times and instead become the dominant. Within these pages, we will look at the many elements involved in being a submissive male and how to get the best out of your experience. Hopefully, by the end of it, you will have a greater understanding of why you personally feel its importance to you and how to achieve your objective of enjoying the role to its fullest.

Chapter Two – Who Am I?

There has been much research about from where our sexual desire emanates. Is it nature or nurture? The answer seems to be a mixture of both.

The consensus is that some sexual arousal is partly innate and utilizes two structures within the brain, namely the amygdala and the hypothalamus. This is the part we are born with and occurs instinctively and without our being aware of its operation. This is called 'cued interest'.

The other part, 'un-cued interest' is developed through early experiences and is at its strongest when we are developing sexually and erotic thoughts prevail. These are obviously going to be much more variable than the cued interests because we are all subjected to widely different experiences and so ultimately we have no control over what turns us on sexually.

It might be something so obvious as being spanked as a child and that corresponded to having erotic thoughts, which continued into adulthood. No doubt that spanking was given by someone who made you feel safe and whom you trusted to show you what was right and wrong.

Also controlled by our brains is the instinct to be either dominant or submissive, or even both, as the circumstances dictate, and both are hardwired into our brains to give us sexual gratification. The expression of, 'expressing his feminine side' may be truer than we first thought on the face of it. We can compare this to the animal kingdom where we see female dogs mounting other females or male dogs mounting other males. The roles can become blurred and interchangeable and produce sexual stimulation.

The biological part in the brain seems to be much easier to explain than its partner. There have been incidences where babies have been born as one gender but for one reason or another have been raised as the opposite sex. Even though the child has not been informed of the circumstances, they have still reverted to the original gender role. One such famous case is that of David Reimer in 1965 who when undergoing circumcision accidentally lost his penis. His horrified parents consulted a famous sexologist Dr. John Money who convinced them that if they operated on the baby and gave him a vagina instead he could be successfully raised as a female. They did this and he was injected with hormones that made him grow breasts and develop womanly curves.

Despite his parents' best efforts however, he rejected everything that was considered to be feminine and instead displayed masculine behavior and traits. No longer able to keep up the charade, when the child reached the age of 14, his parents told *Brenda* that actually he had been born *David*. He was hugely relieved and went on to undergo further operations, which gave him back a penis, although it was non-functioning. He also had a double mastectomy to remove his breasts and eventually even went on to get married. Sadly, at the age of 38 he committed suicide by shooting himself through the head because he was unable to overcome the very successful brainwashing that had been applied throughout his childhood. This clearly indicates that fighting what comes naturally is not a healthy way to deal with sexual inclinations that are regarded as being unwholesome by the general public. The enforced denial of natural instincts in fact is totally unnatural, and an ill-conceived way of attempting to shape everyone to the replicated model of a preferred prototype of the majority.

In a study carried out by Ogi Ogas and Sai Gaddam's *A Billion Wicked Thoughts. What the World's Largest Experiment Reveals about Human Desire (2011)*, they posited that men were turned on by visual representations and women were turned on by romance and stories. For women, sex was more cerebral. This study was done using the Internet so that it allowed people to complete a survey on their sexual preferences allowing them to be completely frank, but this study diverged from previous ones by its anonymity. For that reason, it was regarded as being more honest and probably more accurate than its predecessors. This research validated the assumption that a man is ruled by what's between his legs and it also proved that men have more sexual neural pathways to the brain than women have. As soon as men are presented with visual erotica they are aroused both physically and psychologically. Incidentally, it also came as a surprise to discover that men are more aroused at the sight of an erect penis than women are.

This male one-track mind must be tempered with an explanation that they are wired to view women as vehicles that can be used to propagate the next generation. To ensure this, it is reasonable to suppose that is why man is not essentially monogamous, and so it is an understandable instinct to have developed evolutionally in their brain. Men have neurologically developed to be dominant whereas women are conditioned to instinctively search for a partner who can provide safety and security for herself and her children. Or so it has been historically but now that is perhaps due for redesign to fit in with the Earth's needs.

The report also shows that men are turned on by what they consider to be new and novel, which might explain why they seek new experiences which could sometimes be perceived as being outside the norm, such as being a submissive perhaps. Playing the role of sub opens up a whole new avenue for exploration. This could be a prolonged chapter or a brief interlude but new territory often is more appealing that a path well-trodden and predictable.

Another cue for arousal is a sense of danger and this could be evoked by a sense of difference and because male submission is regarded as taboo by many still in society. This might be because there is a feeling of doing something, which is socially or culturally, regarded as forbidden, perverse and not acceptable by the masses. Just by performing the taboo task alters the physiology by quickening the heart rate, raising the muscular blood flow and making us breathe faster. This is controlled by the sympathetic nervous system, which is also responsible for, surprise, orgasm. This no doubt accounts for the part that fantasies play in our sex lives. Imagining ourselves in perilous situations at which we are at the mercy of someone else can help us to climax. So that would seem to suggest that actually taking part in a physical role play, playing out that fantasy, must be so much more powerful and add enormously to sexual excitement and arousal.

If you confide in a potential sexual partner or close friend and they think you are weird or abnormal, turn that back on them. They are unable to break out of their conditioned harness and are tied down with their own guilt about having a traditional sexual role and unable to break out of it or even think beyond its realms. You are the lucky one because you have given the matter much intellectual thought and should now be fully aware of what excites you and how to get it. Each to his own, and it is probably accurate that you are having a better time than the ones who have settled into a comfortable corner and never dared to move out from it. Leave them with the saying *"Don't knock it until you've tried it!"* And don't give them a second thought. You are on an exciting journey while they dare not even take the first step towards fulfillment.

Relinquishing responsibility to someone else can also be a very effective way of escaping from the normal stresses of life. By passing over the reins to a dominant and submitting to their desires offers release - in more than one sense of the word. It can be a place of safety where the sub becomes helpless and needs the dom to take care of him, reminding him of the safe haven he felt as a child.

There are many physiological reasons for men to wish to adopt the submissive role and this does not just apply to sex, as we'll explore in another chapter. The suggestions given here are not exhaustive but probably some of the most common. These feelings can develop at any stage in life and should never be regarded as being abnormal as long as they hurt no one else.

Matriarchal or matrilineal societies still exist in some parts of the world. In Greek mythology, the legendary Amazon tribe existed entirely of women. They were warriors whose prime concern was war and this tribe was sexualized by many *Carry On* type films. However, societies ruled by women still do exist and they have no doubt evolved out of the need of the land where they were born. They adopted practices that would ensure their continued existence. For instance, in many of these matrilineal societies land and property passes down through the woman. The Mosuo in China is probably the most famous with around 40000 members. Property and lineage are passed down through the woman and the man stays with his own mother. They do not have a word for husband or father and simply go from man to man without marrying. They invite the man to have sex with them or just go to his house to have sex and then move onto the next one when they feel like it. Fathers of the children rarely know who their father is and there is no stigma surrounding this. And amongst many others, lineage also passes through the woman in Judaism. Compare this to our own western society and we start to get an idea of how easily we are controlled to answer the needs of the land.

Perhaps it is not unreasonable to imagine that the physiology of our brains evolves just as other parts of our bodies do over long periods of time. As external influences shape the type of human we need on this planet, hopefully our thought processes will work to control how that is achieved, as well as working the other way too. Sadly, this process normally takes eons to occur. However, if our neural pathways can be built and destroyed by any number of methods, including chemicals and alcohol, then surely it is not too incredible to believe that this is actually possible. Indeed, we may even discover a faster route of achieving any desired outcome. So not only will it be influenced by physical changes within the body, namely the brain, but also by environmental factors exerted upon it. As our knowledge about the human brain grows, so too does our capacity to make changes (improvements?) within it.

Finally, something that we all are capable of controlling immediately is the way we think. It would be unfair to be judgmental of others' sexual inclinations, regarded as perversions by someone on the outside looking in. If you are already a submissive man, thus going against the constraints that the narrow mindedness in a modern western society places upon you, then you should be aware of how punishing opinion can be against your own sexual inclinations. Try to understand others and let them do their own thing. The more open and permissive we all learn to be about sex the easier it is for everyone to lead a healthy and fulfilled life, which is multidimensional. Keep your mind and your heart open and be willing to share your wisdom. Only you know how long it took to acquire it. Let us move out from behind the closed doors and closets where suppression and self-doubt can only lead to unhappiness. I am not professing you take out an ad declaring your sexual inclinations because I think more than one person might find you a nice padded cell. But rid yourself of the feelings of guilt and realize that it is not wrong to want to live out your fantasies; it is instead wrong to deny yourself or anyone else that opportunity.

If it feels good, do it!

Chapter Three - Submissive to Alpha

Being a submissive man does not mean that you have to be submissive in all areas of your life of course. The degrees of submission are on a sliding scale and cover a very wide spectrum. Many men choose to keep it just to the bedroom while for others it may be integrated seamlessly into their day to day household activities. The roles of submissive and alpha are also interchangeable and even during a sex session an individual can flip from one to the other. It's about what the couple feel comfortable with and desire.

Even the heads of multi-million dollar organizations or top politicians may need respite from the daily grind of constantly being in control and having to make decisions that can potentially affect others' lives fundamentally. It cuts across social class and the reasons for have submissive tendencies are remarkably complex.

It might be a surgeon who literally is responsible for making life or death decisions on a daily basis. It is understandable that high powered males who are required to exude an unmistakable air of authority and be the alpha male in their working lives should need to relinquish that responsibility from time to time and escape a very demanding reality. This does not mean that they do not enjoy their profession; in fact, it may mean the very reverse, that they give everything to it and it is emotionally and mentally draining. And relinquishing control to someone that they love and trust is far healthier than resorting to drugs or drink. And far safer.

Being a submissive or living out the submissive role playing may happen very infrequently or it may be a planned event with a partner or entail an occasional visit to a professional domme. It may be different every time or it might be variations on a theme. At first, an alpha male may well struggle with swapping roles, even though he craves to do so because he has been so well conditioned throughout his life into believing that he must always be the strong man and be in charge at all times. Incredibly, should a well-known public figure reveal a sexual preference for being a submissive it still may be a cause for public titillation and it is doubtless a sign of denial in many cases for men who are overtly alpha. It takes courage to come out and admit to yourself what your deepest desires are, especially when everything you have been taught up to now is to be the exact opposite of what you want to do. But it doesn't have to take over your life. Not all submissives have dungeons in their basements and a cupboard full of sex toys that would make a nun faint. It's a question of degree and what suits you personally.

Nevertheless, an alpha male may struggle to let the facade of manliness down but it can be done by introducing subtle changes into normal life. For instance, let's take a hypothetical example. An alpha male may well take inordinate pride in being a breadwinner and providing for his family. It is ingrained into him deeply by a family who were traditional and were not fortunate enough to explore any opportunities, educational or otherwise but had to concentrate on acquiring and maintaining a secure and safe environment for their child. Our submissive male, on the other hand, has had the privilege of a good education by the good grace of his parents, and has the luxury to spend time on self-exploration and forming trusting relationships. He knows himself well, including sexually, and has reached the point where he is ready to put into practice some of his fantasies of male submission.

So far, his orthodox upbringing has perhaps held him back but one day, he picks up a magazine or meets someone at a party and this one day changes his life forever. He decides to take note of the new information that has been presented to him and is determined that he will follow the advice to become himself. His workload is so heavy, he is extremely successful in his field and yet he has been yearning to find a way of seeking some respite from the heavy burden his professional life places upon him. And his search begins. It takes him into new circles where he finds that he has no reason for guilt and that he is not the freak he has feared himself to be. The new knowledge and sight of the lifestyle he wants to acquire are evidence of all things being possible and within his reach.

He is already in a stable relationship with a woman he loves and trusts, so how does he begin to integrate his desire for being submissive? It is not only linked to the sexual side of him but he wants to share a burden of responsibility with his partner. So he makes a plan. He earns enough to take hold of the financial reins but one way of introducing submission into his life is to let his female partner be responsible.

This is something that you might like to introduce into your life but it is entirely dependent on your circumstances and preferences. There is actually a name for this and is it "findom." It might be completely or just in certain areas. You might go to a restaurant for a meal and she insists on paying. Slowly, the idea of sometimes being out of control gently infiltrates your lives together. It might be as simple as you might let your partner choose what to watch on TV, even when you want to watch golf, but you subjugate your own needs for hers and even find you enjoy it and even discuss the program afterwards. You ask your partner to make important decisions for you both and agree to do as she decides, always letting her have the final word. You run a bath for her and help her to undress and dress, maybe rubbing her body down with oil afterwards. The important message is that you do what she wants you to do without question because she is in charge and you do as you are told. You are placing your free will, even if only in certain areas, into her hands.

The distinction between alpha and submissive males can appear as being very distinct but it is rare to find a man who is completely one or the other. It can never be that black or white and all human beings are thankfully multidimensional and have many layers that make them into what they are. Historically, it was always thought that women preferred the strong he-man portrayed in pop romantic novels as being able to make every woman in sight swoon with the heady delight of passion as he took her in his muscular arms and ravaged her. A little woman needed someone who could be constantly in charge of everything and make snap decisions on momentous topics.

In parts of the world, in countries that exist around brute strength and which depend on leaders being autocratic to get what they want, an alpha male leader must be domineering and command respect, earned or not but probably the latter. But studies done by Cheng et al (2010) on university athletes showed that the alpha males within the group were found to have unlikeable characteristics such as being unethical and immoral, narcissistic and generally disagreeable. They were described as not being cooperative or helpful, were not all that popular and in fact were low on self-esteem. By contrast, their prestigious fellow beta members of the team were the ones who took the role of leader and they in turn were described as popular, cooperative, helpful and more intelligent and they had better social skills and higher self-esteem.

This is a clear indication that different attributes are required in different circumstances. For instance, if a giant of commerce or industry, who is at the top of his game, was sent to an overcrowded and violent prison, as a prisoner, he would sink to the bottom of the pile in an environment for which he was ill-equipped to deal and he would have to adapt to survive in a hostile and strange place. Attributes that made him popular would help that survival and this transfers over to civilized societies. A leader must listen to those he governs and take their wishes and needs into account. Otherwise, evoking nothing but negative feelings, sooner or later he will be toppled. And the same rule transfers easily into more personal relationships.

In recent decades male and female roles have blurred around the edges and women welcome the softer side of men, especially in a lifetime partnership where both are responsible for major decisions. Ideally, the relationship is so open and trusting that an alpha male can confide his desires to his partner and they can discuss in depth how far they want to go sexually. Experimentation should be easily facilitated and both partners must feel comfortable with it. Sexual relationships should always be reciprocal, at least to some degree, or there can be little joy for the partner who is getting no gratification from the union.

Sometimes, a submissive male may want to keep this side of his nature apart from his long-term partnership. This might be because he already knows that she would not accept the idea under any circumstances and he does not want to put an otherwise perfect relationship to the test by insisting that she takes on the role of domme in the sexual side of their relationship. Or it could be that doing it secretly adds an extra frisson of danger and magnifies the experience and heights of sexual gratification and pleasure. Everyone's circumstances are different and you must find your own level that makes you feel comfortable and happy, ideally without hurting or deceiving a partner. You know your own circumstances best and no doubt you will consider them carefully before risking everything for what could be classed as 'a bit on the side'. Cheating on a partner should never be acceptable under any moral compass in any kind of relationship. Ask yourself how you would feel if you found out someone was cheating on you behind your back. A later chapter is dedicated to this subject.

Fundamentally, self-awareness is paramount. Should you decide to explore this part of your psyche for the first time and you have always considered yourself to be an alpha male, you should consider why you feel the need to do so. What is it that excites you about this sexual foray? The answers can be extremely illuminating and lead onto enormous leaps of self-knowledge, which can enrich relationships and sexual enjoyment.

Think about two gay men in a relationship and how they may well find role adoption of sub and dom much easier to adopt than a heterosexual couple who have assumed traditional roles. Gay men are used to having to adopt the role of alpha in certain environments, especially in their professional lives but maybe to their families too, even though it may go against the grain. After a while, it should become automatic. After all, we all adopt many different *hats* for different situations -

that is we react differently within each group we may belong to, be that work, home, family, social etc. Everyone we know knows a different me.

What you show yourself to be in your professional life need not be the sum total of who you are. It may be part of what attracts a women to you but then, like any other relationship, there has to be different aspects to explore within that relationship. Like any other union between two people, it is about a shared sense of values and an ability to find common crossover points where you can identify and empathize with each other. This is a step on the route of the alpha male sharing his submissive side and it is up to the couple involved how far they want to travel that route. To find out then you must discuss it and find a level that suits you both. You don't have to jump in with both feet; in fact it could be totally terrifying to suddenly produce a set of handcuffs and a whip instead of the normal bunch of flowers you might present your partner with. Talk about it first.

Of course, it's always about balance. Most people will respond to another person who is kind and responsive, interesting and interested. The two roles of alpha and beta can cross over at numerous points and this might be across the professional and personal arenas. Most men - and women - will be a mixture of these two and even if your profession calls for a level of dominance, different facets of your personality can still be introduced alongside to foster a feeling of empathy and cooperation. You are in charge of the role you adopt and that goes for all areas of your life. There is no concrete rigidity of how you adapt along that spectrum. Learn to be confident in your own skin and go for what you want and what makes you and your partner happy. Don't be afraid to show your feminine side either because that soft and gentle persona will always be acceptable by everyone you meet. If it isn't, it's their problem, not yours.

Chapter Four – Foundation of a Healthy Relationship

Let's be real here. Female-led relationships are rare, and this gives both submissive men and dominant women very few resources to refer to. There isn't a formulaic approach to building the perfect FLR. And because it's not as common as its MLR counterpart, this seemingly blurs the lines of boundaries and gives a rather foggy idea of what makes a healthy D/s relationship.

I'm going to dissect this dynamic to explain what I mean. A relationship that is dependent one a party more than the other never lasts. Female-led doesn't mean that women will be the center of your world, where you'll do nothing but serve them and await their appraisal and validation. This is dependence, and it's unhealthy and unattractive to women, which I'll explain in more detail later.

Submissive men do have power in the relationship; it's just channeled in a different manner. You choose to submit, and the moment you opt-out of this dynamic, it stops. There is no (actual) contract that binds you to be a slave or a sex servant. You merely choose to act like one because it turns both you and your partner on. Approaching women with the mindset of filling some sort of void that you have has never ended well. This is never what dominant women seek.

For instance, some men may approach a dom, thinking

that the relationship will involve being taken by surprise with sexual acts that may be done anywhere and anytime. And while, in theory, it may sound hot to pretend to resist sexual intimacy, it's not fun in reality. This is why you need to establish boundaries before you start having sex. Consent is the foundation of your relationship.

Boundaries pretty much include everything. Some couples may want to have a D/s relationship inside and outside of the bedroom. For instance, I've met some men who enjoyed it whenever I ordered them to do the housework for me. You'd think they only get off on dirty washing panties, but even being made to do the dishes satisfies them, because it makes them feel like they're useful to their doms beyond the parapet of sex acts.

Other couples may prefer to keep this dynamic in the bedroom and share a conventional relationship otherwise. This all depends on what you and your partner like, and it's not just something you find out as you go with the flow. If you decide to do something against your will thinking that it's part of the package, you'll grow to resent the relationship eventually. And let me assure you that your female partner would be disgusted to know that you're doing something that you don't want to do. Force is not what makes a D/s relationship. The choice to submit is.

On the other hand, boundaries also make sure that both of you equally enjoy sex. Some men may like feet; others find them disgusting. You wouldn't want to be compelled to indulge in a fetish that you don't enjoy, thinking that it's just the way it is. It's not. You and your partner make the rules. You don't blindly follow kinks you see in pornography unless you both decide you enjoy said kinks. Share your fantasies and see what you're both allowed to do.

You see, just because you're the sub in this relationship doesn't mean that you can't set the rules. That's something you need to do before you initiate sex so that both of you feel comfortable, and equally enjoy the experience. This is why I always view D/s relationships as something that can only be gradually built along with trust. I wouldn't advise men to meet a stranger off a dating app and immediately allow them to immobilize them in bed whilst blindfolded. Female-led relationships, especially when it comes to sex, are based on trust. You must trust the person not to cross the line because it can go downhill very quickly if you do.

Another aspect of a dominant-submissive relationship is openness, but that doesn't come without its own set of rules either. Because let's face it, individuals in the BDSM community are far from conventional, and they're always open to trying new games, even if they're not initially sure about them. It might be fun to try them out, but it may also be difficult to opt-out without coming off as pretending to resist, as part of the game. This is where a safe word comes in handy.

A safeword can be anything bizarre that you normally

wouldn't say in bed. So I'd avoid anything such as no, or please stop because these can all be deemed part of your power-play in bed. Always use a safe word if you ever feel like you're in too much in pain, or if you otherwise feel uncomfortable for any reason during sex. This gives your partner a cue for a "time-out," and she should stop immediately. Some couples also like to use a green/yellow/red system. This way, you can easily allow you, partner, to proceed (green), take it slow (yellow) or stop (red).

That said, I'd like to stress how establishing boundaries is not just limited to doing so with your partner. I've met many men who weren't realistic about what they expected and what they could actually tolerate. You can easily get off to porn, showing men getting their cocks and balls stepped on because, in theory, it's sexy when you're just lying in bed and thinking about it. In reality, it takes some great tolerance to pain to enjoy such acts. When you tell a dom that you enjoy certain kinks, she will naturally presume that you have tried them, and have thus had experienced pleasure from them.

If there's anything you haven't yet tried, but like the idea of, I'd suggest being open to your partner and asking her to be gentle and work her way up by using the green/yellow/red system to see how far you can take it. If the pain is not pleasurable, never be afraid, to be honest about that. It doesn't make you look "vanilla" to be less tolerant of pain than others. Your mistress wants you to enjoy the pain as much as she enjoys inflicting it, so always be upfront about how you feel during your power-play.

Now that the importance of boundaries is established let's move on to something I'd like to stress on, and that's how some men can be needy and mistake that for submissiveness. Surely, your mistress will enjoy being spoiled and being the center of attention...in the right context. Some men grow an unhealthy obsession about serving women, possibly in a subconscious attempt to fill a void. And while I feel bad for them, let me tell you that dominant woman are certainly not your therapists.

A woman will always tell whether a sub is playing along to the power dynamic, or is genuinely obsessed with being around her and having nothing else to do than pleasing her. And let me tell you that she won't like the latter if she senses it. On the other hand, you should always find a community where people share your interests – as in other submissive men seeking mistresses. You need to teach yourself about what the common power dynamic is like, and what it usually entails. Some men approach sub-dom relationships as though they will have no say in the rules. Or rather, they find it easier to do so, which also stems from being needy.

When you initiate a female-led relationship with such an attitude, you immediately come off as a leech. Surely, it's fun seeing someone who genuinely enjoys serving me, but what is the point if they have no other interests of their own? Needy men have as much personality as a brick wall, and that makes them anything but appealing partners to doms. And aside from what women think, it's not healthy for you to pursue such a relationship for validation because it will simply never work, and only means that you're seeking this power-play for all the wrong reasons.

A submissive man initiating a relationship will always propose a consent checklist, and will usually be the one establishing rules about what he's willing to do and the kinds of punishments he's willing to receive. I've known submissive men who weren't big on humiliation and only liked a little whipping on the side. While other men may be into full-blown humiliation, licking toes and being spat on is only the tip of the iceberg. The bottom line is, if you don't want to come off as a leech, always set some ground rules which show that you know what you like and what you're serious about investing in the relationship.

Another thing you might want to work on is your expectations. In your own fantasy, you think of yourself as a slave to your mistress who provides. You're at home with your male chastity belt and leash on, awaiting the arrival of your dom. Once she's there, you're ready to present your body to her whenever she feels like it. In theory, it sounds like a dream come true, but it's also a rather juvenile way of thinking of female-led relationships, primarily because all the realistic details are forgotten.

You will sometimes get sick. She will sometimes be too

exhausted to engage in BDSM play and will go straight to bed. At times, you'll spend a day or two like a conventional couple in a vanilla relationship because one or both of you are sick, tired, or just not in the mood. You're not signing away your soul. You will both still get to choose to opt-out of this dynamic whenever you want to, and that's something I highly advise you to stress on before you start engaging sexually with a dominant woman, especially if you're new to the game.

I always advise men to see their submissive sides of themselves as just that: aside. It's not what makes you; it's not your entire personality. Because when you think of it as who you are, you'll find it increasingly challenging to say no when you don't feel like it. You'll find it impossible to say the safe word even though it's a little too rough for you. And this is all but healthy. You want to be able to tap into character. I understand that submissive men are generally submissive beta males, but that's not what I'm referring to right now.

And that is not to say that power-play only applies to sex. You can still do chores for your dom, and you'd be actively playing along. The point is, whenever you need a break, you're entitled to one. If you find that there is no off button on your power game, then you're in an abusive or a miscommunicated relationship that needs to be fixed or mended.

Now that I've covered everything that could possibly go wrong with FLR let's get to the good part. In my opinion, D/s relationships, in general, are much healthier than their vanilla counterparts. Whether conventional couples realize it or not, the relationship is never equally dependent on both parties in regards to everything. There are always disparities, and there will always be one partner who's more dominant than the other. The difference is, vanilla couples don't incorporate that into their sex lives (as intensely), and they don't really admit the existence of this dynamic.

On the other hand, this is the opposite of how I view FLR in particular. It's an honest expression of who leads, even though both parties fairly contribute to where the relationship goes, and both have control over it. I see this is never successful with vanilla relationships because the power dynamic is not clear, there's always resistance on both ends, and a party usually ends up exerting more effort in the relationship.

When you and your partner have explicitly agreed that you're the sub in the relationship, this allows each of you to know what is expected of you to give and receive in return. Each of you has a role, and each of you exerts equal amounts of effort in the relationship, although you channel it in completely opposite manners.

An FLR is the perfect yin-yang.

That is when the yang likes to get spanked.

In general, I personally find D/s relationships more expressive and much more sensual. Nothing says trust like being tied to a bed blindfolded, unable to anticipate when or where you'll get a whipping next. You trust that your partner will not hurt you, and will only inflict a pleasurable amount of pain. It's exciting. It keeps you on edge, and it's this dirty little secret between you and your partner that no one else knows about.

The idea that people see a completely different person out in the social sphere makes your D/s relationship more special. Only you get the privilege of seeing your partner in full latex with a paddle. And similarly, only she can be intimate with you in such a way. It's sensual and sexy, and it brings couples closer. I think there's something unique about BDSM power play in general that makes couples much more passionate about each other. They tend to grow a spark that lasts because their relationship is always exciting.

I'd also like to reiterate that a healthy D/s relationship can have, according to my own experience and that of others, some mental health benefits. It's hard to come out to people about being submissive, especially when you're a man because they tend to view you differently and associate negative connotations to something that you enjoy in a safe environment. But most importantly, people in vanilla relationships don't realize how D/s couples have it better. You can analyze my sexual tendencies through Freudian theories all you want, but does it matter why I may like these kinks if they're practiced with someone I trust in a consensual manner?

When I talk about healthy D/s relationships, I

inevitably have to bring this up. Are they healthy to begin with, even though some may argue they are only sexual tendencies that stem from child abuse? I wouldn't care too much where they come from, as long as you ask yourself these two questions:

1) Is this consensual?

2) Do I feel safe?

If the answer to both of these questions is yes, then go ahead and do whatever you want. Get slapped and spanked, get your torso stepped on by high-heels before your mistress ties you to a cross and whips your ass. You're a man with unconventional kinks, and you like to be humiliated by your partner in an elaborate sex dungeon. It may sound unorthodox to others, but I'll take consensual, safe sex in a heartbeat if it makes both me and my partner happy. So whoever argues that what you share with your partner can't be healthy, shrug it off and put that leash back on. You don't have to confide in others about what you do in the bedroom if it makes you feel uncomfortable. That's another reason why D/s can be exciting. It's usually secretive, and that makes it all the more fun.

Now that you know what makes a D/s relationship healthy let's take a look at how you may want to incorporate power-play in your everyday life. As I said, some men may enjoy being dominated in the bedroom, while others would be interested in making a lifestyle out of it. I'm going to be demonstrating the latter. Men who seek this kind of relationship can refer to themselves as 24/7 submissives. A fair warning, though; it's not for everyone.

There are oftentimes rules that are made about the kind of clothing you can wear at home. Some women may demand that you wear chastity belts, others may ban boxer briefs or any kind of underwear. You might be required to wear a leash or a full body suit on some days, depending on the rules that you set together beforehand.

When I say that you'll be a 24/7 submissive, it's much more flexible than it sounds. That means that you still have time for work and housework, and you usually incorporate this kind of play in your common free time. For instance, you may be required to put on such outfits as soon as you come back from work. That doesn't mean that you need to prepare yourself for sex daily, because you'll find that it's a little unrealistic for long-term relationships.

Many mistresses also like to tease men. You may be spanked on some nights, teased on others, and you may spend a week or more without intercourse, only edging. It's sexy and makes intercourse much more fun, as it feels like a reward that you've earned. Sex takes time and investment, so teasing is a much sexier way of delaying sex than flopping yourself on the bed and promising your partner that you'll try to be less exhausted tomorrow.

That's another thing I respect about D/s relationships. You schedule everything and set realistic expectations.

Today you get a whipping. Tomorrow, I'll sit on his face while I have a cigarette or two, and on the weekend, I allow him to penetrate me, but only if I'm on top. It's all organized and planned, and it's always different. Sometimes, I may surprise him with a reward that he doesn't expect, and his reaction turns me on. This is what you'll be in for when you date a mistress, and it's equally exhilarating and healthy for both of you.

Generally speaking, if it doesn't feel right, then it probably isn't. What I love about BDSM is how animalistic it is – how it satiates our deepest instincts in the wildest ways possible. Your gut feeling is equally important when you engage in such power-play. If there's anything that makes you feel uncomfortable, always be open about it. Use a safe word or the green/yellow/red system I mentioned above. You'll know that you're in a healthy D/s relationship, and you'll easily see red flags when there are any. Loosen up, and get yourself that mistress.

Chapter Five - It's Not All about Sex

Submission does not just apply to sex of course. A man may choose to be submissive in other ways. Below is a list of suggestions. It's not exhaustive and I'm sure that you could think of many more.

Financial

We touched on financial submission in the previous chapter. This is when a submissive man chooses to let his partner take care of the finances. Whatever he earns may go straight into her bank account or maybe a joint account but he might be given an allowance or has to ask for anything he needs. There are practical and organizational advantages to this as well as emotional. If one person is in charge of the purse strings then all expenses and outgoings should be centralized and under control. This would send out a clear message to the woman in the relationship that her submissive partner trusts her to take care of the important things that matter in their lives such as keeping the roof over their heads and ensuring all the utility bills are paid and not in danger of being cut off. This would be the case especially if he is the only earner in the home. She can become the lady of leisure who lunches while he goes out to work to keep her in the way to which she's become accustomed.

This is a very different scenario to the 1950s when women were 'the little woman at home'. By the 1960s, the bra burning had begun and women fought hard for their equality. What might have been a better goal to aim for would have been supremacy. Because they were not only fighting for the freedom of being able to work and decide when and if to give birth but also for equality in the workplace. For many of them, this meant joining men in the labor force again, at a much lower pay rate, and running a home too. Hardly equality. Even though things are slowly catching up now as far as the spread and share of domesticity and childcare is concerned, there is still a long way to go.

Findom does not have to be as clear cut as the male submissive asking for money as and when he needs it but it can be beneficial in such a way that the couple has to discuss major purchases before one of them goes off at a tangent and spends large amounts without consulting the other. Even by pooling the resources of both earners in a couple, if one person holds the strings then there will be no nasty surprises in store for the other partner and this method should encourage excellent financial literacy in a couple and an organized pattern of regular spending. This does not, of course, mean that common sense has to go out of the window and give license to the female to spend, spend, spend on things only for herself and neglecting essential household bills. So do check in from time to time, just to make sure you have a partner who is totally trustworthy and knows what she's doing.

Housework

It is now becoming more and more common that a man is in charge of the housework rather than it being the sole traditional role for women. Indeed, it might well be that he is the better cook or better at cleaning than his partner. He may enjoy shopping and looking for bargains or treats for them both. This would fit in particularly well when the woman is a full time worker and the man does not work or works only part-time but nevertheless, this doesn't necessarily have to be the case and there doesn't have to be a reason. Quite often, this kind of regimen will occur naturally and evolves over time. Other times it might be agreed by a couple and last for varying amounts of time as decided upon by both parties. This can be on a scale of always making the meals or becoming a domestic slave. So it could range from being sent on errands to being a total domestic slave. Parties within a relationship might agree to swap traditional roles so that a man might do all the household chores and the woman does things like decorating and car maintenance. Sometimes it can be a natural preference and other times it can be an agreed - or enforced - decision between two people.

Parenting and Childcare

For a couple of decades now it is increasingly common to see a man who is responsible for full time childcare. As more and more women enter the professions and their earnings outstrip those of the man, it makes more financial sense for the lower wage earner to stay at home with the children full time while the woman goes out to work and supports the family. This might be because they have decided that the child needs a full-time parent at home to look after them and be responsible for raising them. Or, it could be that the cost of childcare is prohibitive. No doubt this fairly modern trend will have a knock-on effect in line with the way modern economies develop: it could affect how children develop. Alternatively, being responsible for children's welfare and wellbeing full time may alter how the caregiver perceives himself on a more global scale.

Objectifying

This is acting as an inanimate object and serves as a form of humiliation. It might be a piece of furniture for instance so that the male is on all fours and the female rests her feet on his back while she drinks wine and watches TV. Jeff Gord, a bondage artist, called this forniphilia and specifically describes the act of human bodies being incorporated into pieces of furniture. Gord used to extend it to is nth degree and make people part of the furniture so that they would have to stay immobile for long periods. Often they would be gagged and there would be a danger of suffocation so that the submissive's welfare had to be checked regularly. This does not have necessarily lead to sex but could certainly be a method of foreplay and certainly humiliation.

Foot Worship

This is similar to objectifying but the submissive male

would lie on the floor and the domme would rest her foot on his face for long periods. It is common for the Domme to wear stiletto heels in this scenario, which she may use to press into his face or other parts of his body, including his genitals. He could also be told to go on all fours and be made to lick her boots or suck her toes and feet.

Golden Rain

This is allowing your partner to urinate on you and again is a method of humiliation. It can be done onto bare skin or through see through tables so that the urine doesn't have to touch the skin. Some men perceive this act as an honor rather than degradation because the act is so intimate and they are allowed to be part of it.

Acting as a Human Ashtray

Not to the point of stubbing out the cigarette on them, depending on taste I suppose, but as another form of humiliation. A sub might kneel in front of his mistress with his tongue out for instance and she flicks her ash onto it.

Feminization/Sissification

This is when the submissive man dresses up as a woman and acts in a feminine way to appear like a woman or even an exaggerated version of a woman. Going out in public might cause more humiliation - or the sub might enjoy it more! This might go as far as wearing a wig and makeup and dressing in a particularly vulnerable female fashion such as schoolgirl or even in a maid's outfit so that he appears subservient. The man's name may change into its feminine form so Tom becomes Tomasina or George becomes Georgina. He may be given names such as princess or baby or more derogatory names such as slut or whore. Giving relevant chores to the persona make may it all the more humiliating; perhaps they have to answer the door to the postman like this.

Trampling

This is the act of literally walking over someone in an attempt to cause him or her pain or at the very least humiliation. It is most effective when the dom wears stilettos of course.

Verbal Abuse

This might be about the size of the penis or how stupid he is. It is about attacking the ego not destroying his self-worth. It's about stripping back the ego and reducing him to an obedient servant to the woman's will and desires. It should be carried out authoritatively and with confidence so it reaches its full impact and is realistic. Women can enjoy total dominance over their male partners but this does not necessarily mean that they have to be cruel all the time. A man must earn a woman's favor.

Subjugation of Ego

This explanation almost goes without saying because a male submissive wants his needs to be secondary to his partner's. This might be as simple as letting her choose where to eat out or who to see socially, whether he likes them or not. If he doesn't behave appropriately he would be punished for bad behavior. By doing this, the male appears tender and the female should not be afraid that she is being selfish because she is doing what her partner wants her to do. This type of behavior is common to all areas of life which the couple share and should be practiced at all times until it becomes second nature.

Primarily, a submissive man is seeking the loving approbation of a significant female in his life and if she takes control it might stem back to a dominant female from his childhood who was always in charge, but he didn't mind because he always felt safe and loved by that person. Conversely, the dominant woman from his past may never have found him good enough and so he must constantly strive to improve to impress the significant female figure in his life. The dominant female partner takes the place of that significant woman from his past and makes him feel cherished within the boundaries of domination.

Renting Him Out

This is a good way of earning a little extra money. The woman asks friends if they have any non-sexual jobs they want doing such as gardening, decorating - things that her partner can easily manage in his spare time.

However, any money he earns has to be paid directly to the female and a private report given about his work. Freebies could also be offered.

Again, this list is not exhaustive. The objective of the exercise is to ensure that the submissive male hands over any authority of part of it to his partner. This can be in just one area or as many as you can think of. It is primarily about suppression of the male ego and allowing the female to take charge of situations. Try and be creative. Opportunities to exploit this form of non-sexual domination abound in everyday life and it can prove enormously liberating for both parties.

Chapter Six - How to Find Your Dominant Woman

Statistically, submissive men seeking dominant women far outnumber dominant women seeking men to dominate. However, that is not to say it is impossible; in fact, far from it. And there are various way of achieving this.

Personal Ads

The most obvious would seem to be placing your own personal ad but you should be extremely cautious and use a new email address. Your ad should be as appealing as you can possibly make it because you need to attract as many potential partners as possible. You should know what sort of a person you are looking for so that they can identify with what you want, but more importantly you should clearly state what you could offer them. Like any other relationship the other person needs to know if you have anything in common to start with so at least you have something to build on and are not going to be sitting like two dummies when you get together.

When you have exchanged sufficient emails to make you feel comfortable ask for personal details and exchange more photographs. Perhaps you could then progress to chatting online. There are so many ways to do this and I am sure you already have a preference but Messenger and What'sApp are free and you can get to know each other very well through this medium.

Finally arrange to meet but always in a public place for at least two to three dates. Some might argue that meeting someone from the internet is dangerous rather than in a natural situation in real life, but is it really any more risky than meeting someone you have only met once in a social situation or whom you see at work and whom you know nothing about? If you didn't take any risks, then you'd never meet anyone. Just use your head and be sensible. Take things slowly and get to know each other. Be sure you can trust each other and, if meeting for the first time, then leave a trail so that in the event of anything untoward happening, you can easily be tracked down. Have someone call you after a certain amount of time to check that you're okay and have a code to specify that you are - or not. If not, then make your excuses using the call as the reason why you have to leave so soon.

After discussing general things such as work and hobbies, try and discuss in detail what each of you want from the relationship. Is this likely to be a long-term, loving relationship or is it all about sex? Should it be monogamous or are you both free to have other partners? When you have proven yourself to her she may be ready to take it onto the next level but never try and force things. That would not be appropriate behavior for a submissive. If you have started off by placing an ad focusing on a submissive relationship, then bringing up the topic after chatting for a while about more general things is not untoward. Rely on your instincts and you should know when the time is right to bring the subject of sex up. If she seems uncomfortable, then perhaps you have chosen the wrong moment or have been too premature. On the other hand, if you have been specific about what you are looking for, there should be no problem about at least asking how she feels about it in principle. If she backs off completely in horror, then ask if she has had second thoughts and no hard feelings felt.

However, there can be problems using personal ads in that you are using your desire to seek a D&S relationship as your prime focus and motivation instead of meeting someone and building a relationship first, after which you introduce the other sexual elements. In that way, the trust should already be present and you are practicing in a loving and safe environment. On the other hand then, if you are simply looking for someone to share your enjoyment of this sort of sexual titillation, personal ads may be an acceptable way to meet someone and you're both clear from the start that is all you are after. Use it as a way to practice and experiment. At the very least, it can be a pleasant social situation when you can practice your submissive social skills.

Try and let the woman take the lead after you have discussed what you want. If she is experienced, then take this as an excellent opportunity to learn and feel your way along the path to submission. If she is a novice, then you are both learning together and should discuss ground rules and how you will both feel safe. Discussing what you want in detail can be erotic in and of itself.

Make sure that she is aware of any pain boundaries you do not wish to cross; this might need some experimentation so let her know that it is going too far by agreeing on a safe word so she knows she has to be more gentle or stop altogether. The safe word you use should be something that is not part of normal daily conversation such as *giraffe* or *banjo,* something totally obscure. If you simply make the safe word *stop* your partner will not know if you really mean it or not and may have to stop what she is doing to ask you, which could spoil the moment. You will find your own level of tolerance but this does not deter you from trying to please her in other ways. You should be treating your woman like a queen. Listen to her and take note of what she wants and what she needs you to do for her. Do not overstep the boundaries agreed. Every relationship finds its own level and that includes every relationship you are likely to form.

Leave a Calling Card

If the person you want to be with is in your workplace, or perhaps somewhere else you go regularly where there are a lot of people, it might be an idea to test the water before plunging in. It could be part of the game to make it fun. You could have anonymous cards printed which intimate that you are interested in finding a domme and ask that person to leave a relevant sign to indicate if they are interested in getting together. Make sure your cards looks classy rather than tacky. The sign that they leave to show that the feeling is mutual could be a soft toy wearing a blindfold for instance. In fact, there are dominatrix bears readily available on the Internet. If you go in next day and there is a blindfolded teddy on everybody's desk then you know your game is a bit of an office joke so at least you know that the answer is probably no. If, on the other hand, the teddy is on the desk of that special person you could move in and ask that person out.

If the woman is sexually adventurous or up for trying new opportunities at least, she will at least be curious about who has left the card. When you declare yourself, it is up to her to say yes or no. Start by inviting her out for a drink or something else equally innocuous. The woman can tell any curious people who asks what the teddy bear is doing on her desk that she was given the bear by a boyfriend or husband as a joke because he thinks she is a slave driver. While you're out, drop into the conversation that it was you who left the card or that you liked the blindfold on the teddy. You should play it by ear but don't rush at things with all flags flying. Get to know each other a bit better first and then enjoy each other.

Look Out for the Right Woman

This may sound obvious but if you are looking for a domme then you should not be asking out the shy and timid wallflower, however nice she is, at least not when you're just starting out. This sort of partner might be for when you are much more experienced and for that time when you are confident enough you can teach her to be who you want and need. Let's face it, some women are never going to be comfortable playing the domme and you don't want to mar your submissive sexual journey by having the memory of an hysterically upset female trying to escape you.

Look out for assertive and confident women, aggressive even, someone who already feels comfortable about bossing men about. Ask her out and go from there. If she is already dominant, she will most likely be able to tell instinctively that you are subservient and start enjoying taking full advantage of it. Open doors for her, bring her flowers, and treat her like a princess. The relationship should develop naturally when you let her have her own way constantly and always demur to her wishes. Of course, don't let anyone totally trample all over your feelings. You still have needs of your own and although you might enjoy role play and demur to your partner's wishes some of the time, you still should command respect and love. Who wants a fantastic sexual if it is with someone who holds you in genuinely fierce contempt? Relationships should be built on trust and love and even acts of punishment should be meted out with the welfare of the recipient uppermost in the domme's mind. It is about giving you what you want, not necessarily what you deserve. Although of course, these two might well be the same.

Join a D&S Support Group

Most major cities have these now so you are already

starting off in the right place to find someone of a like mind by being a member of such a group. Be prepared to be one of a large and eager queue of men, which outnumbers hugely the number of female dommes who are likely to be part of the group. This ratio is probably representative of the numbers to be found generally so it may well be difficult to meet your special woman. There is also likely to be female submissives there as well as transgenders, plus any other kind of sexual oriented individuals or couples but at least in an environment like this the odds of you finding the right partner are lowered. Try and appear confident and as if you know what you're doing. If the right woman is there for you, she will find you and many happy times will lie ahead.

BDSM or Fetish Clubs

Although these might be regarded as some as being sleazy or tacky, most are far from it. Even if you don't meet *the* one, they are lots of fun and you should bump into lots of interesting and colorful people looking for a great night out. Dress for the part so that you get into role and get ready for an eye-popping, lip smacking night where anything goes. Obviously, there's going to be people of all persuasions here so the more you dress like a submissive the easier it will be for you to attract the right sort of person. Be aware though, your submissive outfit might also attract a lot of attention from gay men so have your answers ready for any unwelcome invitations. And by that, I don't mean that you have to be rude. Most people who attend these sorts of clubs are there for a good time. There will be novices and old timers.

Usually, there is a game room in a fetish club where you will be able to see people attached to all sorts of equipment and receiving their punishing. People don't usually mind if you watch or why would they be there in the first place? If you get lucky, they might even ask you to join in. At the very least, you are likely to have the time of your life. There is also usually a bar and a dance floor. Just be careful whom you leave with and make sure someone knows about it. Have your wits about you and be very clear about what you want. You don't want to be found floating down the river the next day with a plastic bag on your head! Not that this happens as far as I am aware (joke!).

When you have made a fair few new contacts, you might be able to narrow them down into a group of only submissive men and dominant women. You could invite them to a party either at your own place or hire somewhere out and charge admission. Tell everyone to dress up in appropriate clothes. Perhaps you could ask someone to provide entertainment by being strapped down and used for pleasure or just maybe a male strip show. It's your party.

Visit a Professional Domme

If you can afford it, treat yourself to a session - or two - with a professional domme. This is an excellent way of experimenting with what you want and you are literally learning from an expert so it would be money well spent. If your first experience is not up to your expectations, don't be put off. Make sure that you ask her to fully explain what is likely to happen before actually doing it. Ask her about the full range of services on offer and if any appeal to you then you can ask to try them out. You can also experiment with your threshold of pain level. The first one might not be right for you so move on to someone else. No-one's feelings can be hurt when you are paying for a service and you are paying for not just satisfaction but a lesson too. Think of it as finding an instructor, like you would for any other thing you needed to learn: driving, playing a guitar. Sometimes, it matters very much who your teacher is. But at the very least, it's a good night out and probably one you will never forget!

Home Grow Your Own

This is probably the best method. Find a woman with whom you are compatible and build the trust before introducing your submissive desires. You could start showing your submissive side in a non-sexual way to start with by offering to make dinner or fetching coffee or putting her feet up to rest. The ways to give your partner a treat are boundless. When she starts to demand that you do things for her, open up and say that you want to try something a little different because you like her being in charge and that you want to cater to her every whim. Learning as a couple can be fun but she might just surprise you by taking to her new role as domme like a duck to water.

You could try taking her to a fetish club if she's up for it. This would certainly spice up your sex life and you only have to take part in the things you choose to. It might give her and you some ideas though. Of course, it might be that your partner is already sexually adventurous within your partnership and that things have become rather predictable. Introducing voyeurism into the relationship can certainly heat things up. Going somewhere like this is a good way of gaining new inspiration. Get her to put you on a lead and make you go down on all fours when you get there. Maybe you could have your drink served to you in a bowl and have to lap it up at her feet. Maybe you could dress very appropriately as well.

Internet Dating

Look out for specific sites out there and get to know someone online first. Preferably, you want to find someone close to home because even though you can conduct an S&D relationship long distance, it is so much more difficult. If you can't find one you like, then you could always start your own. You could do this on social media sites. There are lots already on Facebook for instance and if it's yours, it can be geographically sited. You're free to make the rules then of what can and can't go and you get to screen everyone who wants to be part of the group so you also get first pick.

Get Out There!

Widen your chances of meeting someone. You'll never meet anyone sitting on your couch, watching TV and just wishing. The more people you meet, the better the chances of you meeting someone who fits the bill. Join night classes where women are likely to be in abundance or exercise classes like Zumba or whatever the flavor of the moment happens to be. Learn something that will come in useful in your new role such as massage. Be friendly in public places, friendly not weird, but there's no harm in smiling and wishing someone 'Good morning'. There might just be an instant attraction that makes you click.

* * *

Finding the dominant woman of your dreams is a little challenging without a dating app or website. The rapid growth of the BDSM community has made it possible for individuals to find the right match for them through designated apps like Fetlife and KinkD. And while these services can make your life easier, they rarely ever tell you how to successfully set up a profile that attracts the right partners.

I've personally come across many dating profiles that immediately turn me off, some of which just try too hard to explain the obvious in simple terms that could have been a little cleverer. Coming across a profile with a bio that says nothing but "Looking for a sexy woman to dominate me" makes me immediately look elsewhere. You're on a Fetish app; you don't need to state the obvious. So without further ado, let me cut to the chase about how you can set up an attractive online profile in a way that makes you stand out.

Mystery

No one likes walls of texts in the bio section. You need to leave a little to talk about with your future mistress. The sexiest part of a healthy sub-dom relationship is building it up; getting to know your dom as you slowly establish a bond. If there's anything I encounter more often than not, it's men who tell rather than show in their bios. "I'm a funny man who knows how to make a woman happy."

Let *me* be the judge of that.

If you want to come off as someone with a good sense of humor, make your bio funny. Impress me by writing something clever and catchy; and at the same time, something that actually says something about your personality rather than what you enjoy. Surely, these dating websites are basically a gateway for fun casual sex, for the most part. But that doesn't mean that dominant women want to get straight to it. They'll want to get to know you, see if you click, before they decide they're going to annihilate you in bed. Or in their mini sex dungeon.

Photos

My least favorite part of dating profiles is when they use stock images of submissive men, or photos of handcuffed wrists. Stock photos aren't going to get you anyone, so always upload photos of yourself.

While sexy photos can be fun, you don't necessarily

have to upload a picture of yourself in bondage to appeal to women. In fact, if it's a casual photograph, which leaves plenty to the imagination, that usually makes it more intriguing and a little more mysterious. Finding someone who suits you should never be stressful and doesn't require a professional photoshoot of you tied to a canopy bed. Be and look natural, and women will likely pick up on your submissive tendencies just fine.

Oversexualization

You're on a kink dating website, which is already sexualized enough. Even the most dominant women want to save themselves the hassle of running into creepy men who only see them as sex objects. That said, most of us wouldn't care if you upload photos of yourself butt-naked as long as your bio isn't overly vulgar, no matter what your intentions are with potential matches. Either upload casual photos with a kinky bio, or the other way around.

Don't let your profile make you look like you're a premium user on a porn website.

If you want to include something sexual that you enjoy doing, tuck it in somewhere in an otherwise decent paragraph. It's random, it's cute, and it makes you seem more empathetic and less of a sex addict.

Self-Centered Bios

This goes for both your bio and your interaction with

any woman you meet on a dating app. Dominant women aren't tools for your pleasure. An FLR is a mutual bond, where each party contributes to pleasuring the other. Don't inundate your profile with things that you enjoy being done to you, because that will make you come off as a man who's only seeking his own pleasure.

Doms will order you to eat them out, suck on their toes, and fuck them; and if you don't appear like you'd enjoy that, then what's the point? While I've initially advised you to avoid making it about yourself, I would also add that you keep it simple and subtle. Don't give off too much information about what you like, and leave some space for you and your potential match to converse.

Research

Porn mostly caters to men, so if your knowledge in sex is based on what you've seen in adult films, then it's all based on male pleasure. Women in those films may seem to enjoy doing nothing but slapping cocks and teasing balls, but in real life, women like to get something in return as well. Look up forums that cater to women; see what dominant women enjoy and what kind of pleasure they like receiving.

That's what you should include in your bio and in your interaction with your matches. A woman who expresses interest in you will go out of her way to ask you what you enjoy, so you don't need to make your kinks the center of the interaction.

To sum this up, let's demonstrate what an unattractive profile looks like. Below is what would turn women away:

- Stock photos/No Photo

- Extremely long bio

- Self-centered bio; for example, "I enjoy being whipped and having my balls tied."

- Overly suggestive bio; for example, "Here for hookups. Let's meet up and fuck!"

On the other hand, here's what dom women would likely look for:

- Multiple photos of yourself

- A clever bio that shows some personality other than just sex drive.

- A bio that makes it about women; for example, "I'll do whatever you tell me and accept punishment when I fail to do so."

- Some room for mystery in the bio

I suppose there is no right and wrong way to set up a profile, just an ineffective and more effective way to do it. By following these tips, you're much more likely to make matches. I'd also advise you to target fetish apps and stay away from generic dating apps like Tinder or OK Cupid, because you're less likely to meet doms there.

Chapter Seven - Communicating Your Needs

Adopting the lifestyle of a submissive man does not have to be all or nothing. It is all a question of balance and if you are in an excellent relationship but where you cannot entirely embrace this role, you have to ask yourself if being a submissive is worth jeopardizing an otherwise perfectly ideal relationship. It's something you should know definitely before putting everything on the line. But you should also know: it is not all or nothing and there can be compromise so that both parties get what they want and are happy providing there is sufficient communication.

If you are lucky enough to be in a happy and established relationship, it is probable that you are already conversant with your partner's sexual desires and proclivities. But after a while, most sexual relationships settle into a pattern and without stepping outside of the habits you have formed as a couple, sex can become boring and predictable, something just to get through for the woman especially. Being a submissive man does not have to dominate your life (hah! wordplay!). No one wants to share his or her lives with a complete doormat so it is important that you find a level and work this out between you. Having an exciting and adventurous sex life will take you down many paths if you allow it to. Being a sub might be just one of those adventures.

Thankfully, we have been given the gift of speech and

so this should, in theory, make it easy for us to express to our partner what we want. But despite that many still struggle to open up and simply lay it on the line. If you find talking about it naturally difficult, it might be a good idea to write down questions that you want to give your partner the answers to. I have set out below a suggested list of questions, which you could print off and hand over to your partner at a prescribed time. Feel free to add any of your own because there is no one who knows you better than you, hopefully! It also includes suggested gestures, which can be used associatively with your partner asking the questions and your psychological processing of the answers alongside. This should be done when you are both fully relaxed and feel comfortable and in a place where a sex session could easily be the culmination, that is on a couch or bed.

You are about to open up and tell her your deepest desires but it will be done using a process of questioning and your answers should be as lengthy and informative as you can make them. Do not be afraid of showing emotion. Laying yourself open can be a deeply moving experience for both of you. Showing her a side of you that she wasn't aware of can bring you even closer together. You are doing this exercise to explain to her at length why this type of sex excites you and so that she fully understands how that instinct has evolved within you. Firstly, you should be naked. Ask your partner to dress in a dominant and sexy outfit and find a comfortable place, resting your head in her lap. Tell her not to reprimand or challenge you if she hears anything that she doesn't like or agree with; that can be tackled later and punishment meted out as required. The object of this exercise is so that you can convey to her how and why you are feeling like you do. It might be a good idea to read the first part of the chapter to her so that she can ask you any questions of her own about the process before you begin on the questions proper.

This is only a suggested list. Something to get you started. Add or subtract those you feel inappropriate to your life's story.

1. When was your first orgasm?

2. How old were you?

3. What made you climax?

4. Who were you with? Describe them.

5. Was your mother responsible for your discipline?

6. Did she ever spank you?

7. How did you feel about it when it happened?

8. Was she ever over-dominant?

9. How did that make you feel?

10. Did you have sisters?

11. Were they dominant towards you?

12. What about other females in your life? Were they dominant toward you?

a) Grandmother

b) Aunt

c) Teacher

d) Nanny

13. Have you had a lot of girlfriends?

Why have you had so many/few?

14. What sort of woman attracts you? Is she demure or raunchy?

15. Why do you prefer that sort of woman?

16. Describe in detail your first sexual experience?

17. Was it a good experience and if so what did you like about it?

18. Was she dominant at all? Or did you have to take the lead?

19. How did you feel about that?

20. What sort of thing excites you most?

21. Tell me about your fantasies in detail. Which is your favorite?

22. Why does that excite you?

23. Do you have any fetishes?

24. Would you like me to wear leather/lace/PVC?

25. What would you like me to do to you?

26. Have you ever told anyone that you want to be dominated by a woman?

27. Did you ever get to that stage with a woman?

28. If so, how did it feel?

29. If I want to dominate you, will you let me do it totally and submit to me   entirely?

30. Would you like to experience pain our sessions? If so, describe it. To what level?

31. In what areas of your life are you willing to submit? Sexually? Financially?   Totally?

32. Would you like me to spank you or whip you?

33. Do you want to be publicly humiliated?

34. Do you want me to verbally abuse you?

35. Do you want to be forbidden to orgasm? Totally?

36. If you trust me, tell me your deepest secrets, the things you have never told anyone else before.

37. When do you want us to start doing this?

38. What would your favorite sex toys be?

39. What would you like to wear for these sessions?

40. What would you like me to wear for these sessions?

No doubt you will answer, "Straight away," and you can get started instantly. Remind her before you start that she should start off in the dominant mode, squeezing your balls or stroking your penis but then when she is asking more probing questions to soften up so that you feel safe opening up to her. You might feel that some of these questions do not apply to you and are not relevant but each suggested question reveals something important about you to your partner.

Perhaps she could write a list of questions for you too so that information is a two-way road. And so is the reciprocal pleasure.

This exercise is as revealing as you both want it to be. However, I would suggest that if you feel safe you are as honest as possible. There is no point lying about how you feel or you are taking a step backwards rather than towards what you want. She might deviate from the questions if you should say something that she does not fully understand and that is fine as long as you come back to the list and keep on track. Agree before starting on the questions that if either of you feel uncomfortable it is okay to stop but that you must give a reason for you doing so. Otherwise, the exercise will create more problems that it alleviates. This is about enlightenment and sharing so only honesty is allowed. Saying that, try not to be brutal and say something that is so hurtful you will never be able to retract it or move past it. Hopefully, you know each other well enough at this stage to know that you must treat each other with respect and that your partner's feelings are important to you.

Chapter Eight - Start Slowly

Okay, you've made the decision that you want a dominant female partner and you want to play the role of submissive. You might have analyzed why you feel like this or maybe not. It's not essential that you do but self-awareness is always useful because if you do not know why you feel like this, how will you explain it to any potential dommes? We've discussed how you would find a partner who is in accord with what you want to do but how do you get started, especially if you're both novices?

You might already have ideas going around in your head - and they might have been there for some time already - but now you have bitten the bullet and decided to go for it. Of course, it depends on your circumstances as to where you will start but let us assume for this example that you are starting off from scratch and that you and your partner are learning the ropes, perhaps literally, together. If you're lucky enough to have found a partner who is totally sympatico then you are already streets ahead but for our purposes here we will use a brand new partnership, neither of whom has any sexual knowledge of each other.

So, it's your first date and you have persuaded your lady to come out to dinner with you. You bring her flowers and compliment her on how lovely she looks. Be attentive and open doors and pull out her chair. Let her choose where she wants to go and ask for her opinion about what she thinks you should eat and drink. Make sure that you have taken care of the transport and never interrupt her when she speaks. Always defer to her superior opinion and advice. In short, be subservient and eager to please. You are in the process of setting the scene and preparing the way ahead.

It is a good idea to get to know each other well first if you are looking for a long-term relationship and this is not just about what you are seeking sexually. In this way, you are building trust in each other. It's about finding out what you have in common and if you have the same sense of humor and values. You should be able to assess whether this woman is already a dominant because she will be self-assured and confident, expectant of your chivalrous behavior because she is used to being in charge and getting what she wants. If she seems shy and timid, this does not necessarily mean that the relationship is a non-starter. There is no reason that this person cannot learn to love being dominant but it will probably take more time to get to where you want to be. Take your time and enjoy yourselves and listen to what she has to say.

Over time, you can open up. If she is a skilled communicator you will find yourself telling her things you have never told anyone before. There are people out there who just seem to have a perfect knack of extracting the most intimate information from you and it can be almost cathartic. If she is truly empathetic she might be able to help you towards the path of self-analysis and may even share some of your hypotheses and have ones of her own to share. You are in the process of building a strong relationship, brick by brick so lay a firm foundation.

Gently introduce the topic of your desires to be a submissive and that you are seeking a domme. Talk about the sort of things you like sexually but please choose the right time and place. Unless the sole purpose of your meeting is sex then it might be unwise to introduce this topic in its fullest depth very early in the relationship. You're out for dinner and say, "More wine? And I would like to be tied up during sex." NO! Wouldn't you run a mile too? And she would probably be laughing as she ran. Or screaming.

By the time you do get into more detail, you may or may not have had sex together but it should be getting easier to talk about your sexual preferences. Perhaps you could suggest watching a raunchy movie together or leave books on the topic of S&D lying around. If she asks about it, offer to lend it to her and say it's something that you're turned on by. Show her the Internet sites you've visited. These don't have to be pornographic but are maybe informative and help to answer questions that she or both of you have. If she does make any attempt at being dominant, obey her. If you laugh or demean her attempts it could mean she will never try again. Tell her how lucky you are to have found her and that she is your queen. Build up her confidence and show her she has complete control over you.

You could shop online for some fun sex toys to try out. Make it fun; it doesn't have to be deadly serious. You could start off with a butt plug perhaps which she inserts and orders you to leave in during sex or until she 'has finished with you.' It should be something you both enjoy and when she sees you are enjoying it so much, hopefully she'll want to continue to please you. And in return, you must be willing to do anything she wants that pleases her. Remember, it's not about just one of you getting pleasure, you should both be gaining from this experience or one party is going to want to drop out of it sooner or later. Don't turn your basement into a dungeon after the first conversation because that might just be overkill. In the early stages, plan sessions together always allowing room for her to be creative in her own ways too.

Decide on a safe word. When you're starting out, she might not realize how far is too far. If she is spanking you for example make sure she knows where to spank you which is on the fleshy part of your buttocks and just at the bottom of them. A cane might be a bad idea to start with because they can cause a lot of harm and she is probably not aware of her own strength yet.

Discuss whether you want to flip from one role to another. She might be role-playing at being a domme to please you and even though she might actually enjoy it, she might still prefer being the sub so make sure you take turns if that is what she wants. It's about experimentation and being absolutely clear about what you both want. Being flexible with what you submit to doesn't mean you have to not enjoy it but if you definitely do not wish it to happen make that clear because there can be a fine line between the two.

Communication is the key and you should both decide if male submission is going to be something that you introduce into every sexual session or just now and again. She might want to save it for special occasions to treat you. Talk about whether you would like to involve others and how to do it. You might already know someone or you might choose to visit clubs that have a sexually oriented theme and where you are likely to find other like-minded people.

Some couples enjoy the cuckold scenario when the man has to watch his partner having sex with another man. This might include being tied to a chair beside the bed or even watching a film of it afterwards if it feels more appropriate. This could be combined with punishment afterwards. The man might even have to prepare the woman for sex with the other man by shaving her pubes for instance and applying her nail and toe varnish. He could help her dress tying her into a tight bodice and putting on her stockings. Even brushing her hair would be erotic if they both knew she was being prepared for another man. Of course, this will not be for all couples but can bring some closer together and it's up to you both to decide if this is what you'd like to try. If it does appeal, there are all sorts of ways that you can develop this. For instance the man might have to help getting the man getting undressed on arrival and maybe he could massage him, including giving him a hand job. The man could even be blindfolded during the sex and perhaps allowed to watch a film of it afterwards as a special treat, if he is good that is.

It might be useful if, after every session, you discuss between you what you particularly enjoyed and what did nothing for you. In this way, as you become more experienced between you, she knows what to do to turn you on and those that's she wasting time on. Even the act of talking about it can be quite erotic. You could also engage in phone sex when she tells you what she is going to do to you when you get home. She could say that you are going to be punished for leaving without kissing her that morning and describe in detail what will happen when you get home. Try and take the call in private because it could be very embarrassing to get up from behind your desk at work for instance with a huge erection saying that you have to get home quickly as you run out of the door.

Buy her gifts, including outfits she can wear, and treat her as your superior and make her feel cherished and adored. Most importantly, have fun and lead a fulfilling and sexually exciting life.

Chapter Nine - Role Playing

Now comes the fun part! Literally. No doubt you have your own fantasies to enact but here are some ideas, which, in turn, may give you some new ones. As mentioned previously, the fantasy might remain the same every time or you might choose to vary it and do something entirely different. Things can be spiced up a little by wearing outfits, which can be rented or you can improvise and make your own. And try your best to get into character or you might just end up laughing all the way through it which although it is a lot of fun won't have the desired effect of fulfilling your sexual fantasies.

You might choose to start with something tame and build up so that it gets raunchier as you go along. You might find that you are both exceptionally turned on by the experience or that you move at a different pace, so try and make allowances for each other and adapt to each other's rhythm. As you know, rhythm is especially important when it comes to most sexual acts.

Because you have discussed at length what sort of things you both want to explore, you have already set boundaries so things shouldn't get out of hand. If you do feel unsafe, that is that this is not for you at all, then remember your safe word and say it, loud and clear. The nature of the beast probably demands that you will feel in peril at times, especially if you have set out that corporal punishment will be doled out, that's exactly the name of the game. Right? You are supposed to feel a sense of fear and scary anticipation.

The following examples are just that. They are loose suggestions, which can be varied as, and how you wish - or how your partner wishes. As long she knows what you like, then she can of course take you by surprise and introduce her own ideas, which will probably by more exciting for you both anyway. First of all, take turns to read through the fantasies below and discuss them together saying which ones turn you on even breaking things down and saying why particular aspects of the fantasy excite you. You could take parts from all of them or incorporate just parts of any of them into your own fantasies. Hopefully, this will get you in the mood immediately or you could plan something special for the week-end or whenever you are both free to spend time together uninterrupted and have a good time.

It might be a good idea for your partner to invest in some garments in a sexy material such as leather, PVC, latex or lace, whatever turns you - and her - on. Perhaps you could get some accessories too such as a dog collar and lead. Improvisation can go a long way so have things you can use as ties and blindfolds. You can use leather belts or household objects. Be creative and use your imagination - both of you. I have written these fantasies from the point of view of your partner because she is likely to be in charge most of the time. But this is a chapter you should perhaps share because it is up to your partner to take the lead in these fantasies. In fact, it might be a good idea for you both to share the entire book.

Sex Slave

This is quite a common one so probably a good place to start. Wear your sexiest and most dominant outfit. Leather always goes down well as does stockings and high leather boots. Perhaps you could round this off with crotch less pants or a thong and a basque, which exposes your breasts. If you have a peaked hat that would finish off your outfit nicely. Wear red lipstick and apply makeup that makes your eyes look dramatic. If you don't possess a whip already, use a leather belt instead. Be inventive, it might be a spatula or a fly swat, which would be particularly appropriate to make him feel as demeaned as you can muster. Now you must pick something - anything - that your partner needs punishing for. This might be leaving the bathroom in a mess even after you have told him constantly about it. Without saying anything leave the room and go the place, which you intend to use for his punishment and get into your gear. When you are ready, and have prepared the scene, get him to join you, either by calling him if he is within earshot or call him on his cell phone and tell him where to find you. If he refuses, then show him how angry you are and tell him it is of extreme importance that he comes.

The sight of you in your sexy get-up should make him gasp. Now approach him using your sexiest hip swaying walk and holding a tie behind your back. Go up to him and kiss him deeply. As you do so take hold of his wrists and put them behind his back. Desist kissing him, walk around him and tie his hands behind him. Secure him firmly so he is unable to move to resist you, you could tie him to a chair, which is already set up for him to take a seat. He has to sit and listen to what you intend to do to him. If he tries to escape, slap him.

Now you have to tell him why you have tied him up so you say that you are going to punish him because that seems to be the only thing that will get the message across and through his thick head that he must clean up after himself. Tell him that you are going to cut off his clothes. If he protests, slap him hard across the face again and repeat until he promises to stay quiet. He is to remain completely naked for the whole of your time alone together; hopefully this can be for a whole weekend.

Tell him that after you have meted out some physical punishment, he will then go, at the end of a lead, the end of which you will hang onto, and proceed to clean the bathroom. When it is cleaned to your satisfaction, he will be allowed to undress you and bathe you. When you have laid in a nice bubble bath, he will fetch you Champagne - or the tipple of your choice. He is to stand with his back to the wall and watch you masturbate. When you are finished, he has to help you get out of the bath and dry you off with a warmed towel. Tell him to clean the bathroom again and then stay there until you call him. You go to the bedroom and dress in your domme gear again and then call him to you. Tell him to bend over the bed just because you want to hurt him again to make sure that he really has got the message. When you have finished, tell him to stand up and you sit on the edge of the bed with your legs open. Tell him that him that he is allowed to suck on one of your breasts and then just when he is starting to enjoy it, tell him to stop. Lie back on the bed with your legs open and instruct him to lick you and make you come. Then turn round and kneel beside the bed and tell him to mount you. When you are satisfied, tell him to go and prepare some food for you and come and tell you when it is ready. Tell him that he will be punished if it is not to your satisfaction.

Keep on in this fashion for the whole of the weekend, using him to do exactly what you want. Make him sleep at the side of the bed and secure him to the bedpost using the lead or the belt. He must sleep completely naked.

Now you are ready to start the process by cutting off his clothes.

Strict Boss

You are the sort of boss who thinks men are useless, very much like your female counterparts, and only employ the token male because the law says that you have to be fair. You treat them with contempt and they have no alternative but to accept your unwritten terms because there is such a shortage of jobs for men and so they have to do their very best to please you. You are dressed in a business suit and from the outside look very proper. You wear very high heels though and silky or fishnet stockings. Your makeup is immaculate and your lips are red. You call your employee into your office for his annual appraisal. You sit behind a desk or table, which should have a clipboard so that you can make notes. The only other chair in the room apart from yours is not around the table. Use a bell or some kind of buzzer to tell him to come into the room. If he does this without knocking, tell him angrily to get out and do it again. Ask him how he has the audacity to be so informal with you.

Explain that he has to stand throughout and that you are going to ask him a number of questions on which you will mark him. If you do not like the answers, there will be consequences. Tell him that you know that he has to do whatever you want or his job is in danger. Ask him if he is still in agreement with that because he did accept it as a condition of his employment with your company. Now start the questions. They should be as out there as you can make them so he has to give answers that you will not accept. Ask him if he has now realized that women are superior. Does he like it here? Does he get on with his colleagues? Ask him if he thinks he should be allowed to stay with the company. What can he do to make sure that you are happy with him? Is he willing to be on call whenever you want him? You can make up your own questions here which will probably be more personally titillating. Every time he gives an answer, note it down and make him wait. At the end of the questions, say you are going to add his marks up and if they fall below 20, he will be below the required scale and have to make up for it immediately. Of course, he fails miserably so you ask him to strip off until he is completely naked. Stand up and go round the desk. If he is not erect, lift his penis up with a pencil and snort. Make a derogatory comment such as, "I see you fall short in that area too." However, it is more likely he will be erect so take a ruler and measure it and then make the same comment before tapping his penis with the ruler. Order him to lock the door or put something against it so that you cannot be disturbed. Tell him to undress you. When he removes your business suit, you should be wearing very sexy underwear, keep your shoes on. Tell him you are going to punish him for his poor work and his stupid answers in his annual appraisal. Tell him that you will not have to monitor him on a much more frequent basis (choose your own) to ensure he is improving, at least in some areas. Tell him to go to the cupboard/drawer and fetch the paddle you use especially for such occasions. Tell him from now he must address you as Mistress. When he brings back the paddle tell him to lean onto the desk and then start whacking him. Hopefully you have enough privacy so that you can make him whelp. When his ass is good and red, tell him to kneel in front of you and thank you for the experience. If he forgets to address you as Mistress, give him some more punishment. Now sit on the edge of the desk with your legs splayed and tell him to crawl over to you. Invite him to show you what else he can do and that it had better make you very happy. When he has made you come, tell him that you haven't quite finished with him. Insert a butt plug into his anus and tell him that he must not remove it for the rest of the day. You will be checking from time to time that it is still there and he must remain naked so that his superior female colleagues are free to do the same. Tell him that he must clean the building to make up for his shortcomings in other areas and that you will call him back later to teach him a lesson that he needs to learn. Allow him water and a small break but watch him eating as if it disgusts you. Throughout the day, call him back into the 'office' and check that his butt plug is still there. If it isn't, give him more punishment. Later, when you are happy that the house is clean, call him back for the lesson. You should have invested in a strap on dildo, which he should watch you putting on. This should be over your sexy underwear or if you prefer just in your stockings. When you have it on, tell him to lean over the desk for his final lesson and after oiling it up start pumping away at him. When he comes, tell him he is disgusting and to go and clean himself up and come back to you. Okay, one last task. He must make you orgasm before he is allowed to finish for the day. Give him strict instructions to do whatever you enjoy most. When you are satisfied, dismiss him but remind him that you will be calling him back at regular intervals to check on his progress. If he doesn't improve, then the punishment is likely to get much, much worse.

Hostage

You have been asked to look after a hostage who is being held for ransom from a rich and powerful family.

He has never known any hardships so you are determined that you will teach him a few lessons of your own. Dress in combats if possible and try and wear a mask over your eyes. The only concession to femininity should be the bright red lipstick and the sexy underwear you are wearing underneath. You could start the roleplay by picking him up in some dark alley or car park and putting a bag over his head. Make sure there are no cameras or you'll soon be seeing some blue lights flashing (or we hope you should!). Splash out and buy some handcuffs, which you should snap on him quickly before bundling him in to the back seat of your car. Drive home and get him in the house without anyone seeing. If you have a basement, take him down there, otherwise, maybe you could keep him in the garage. When you have him back, undress him, still with the bag over his head. Laugh at the size of his penis as you grab hold of it roughly and squeeze it hard. Put a belt around his neck and make it tight enough so that he cannot move. An easy way of securing him would be to put one of the holes over a simple hook. Squeeze his balls hard and then explain that he has been brought here until his father pays you $4m. In the meantime, whether or not his father pays up, you intend to have some fun with him and he is going to find out what it is like to be under the complete surrender of a woman. Ask him if he understands and tell him that to start with he is going to receive a beating, which you are going to take great pleasure in administering. If you have a whip use that, otherwise use a belt and start whipping him on the fleshy part of his butt.

Next you could throw a bucket of cold water over him, which should get rid of any erection that might have popped up. Give his balls another squeeze. Tell him that you are going to inspect him and make sure he is clean before you use him for another purpose. Park his butt cheeks and insert your finger and wiggle it around to arouse him. Tell him you are happy that there is nothing there so far and then put in a butt plug. Spank him a bit and ask him if he is going to be a good boy. Tell him you have not gagged him because he is going to need his mouth but that if he tries to call out for help he will suffer beyond imagination. Put some nipple clamps on him to start with and a cock cage if you have one (always be sure to check out the size is appropriate). Take the bag from his head. You could shine a lamp into his eyes so that he is disoriented and blinded by the flash. Let his eyes become accustomed until they fall on you and then slowly start to undress until you are standing there in all your fantastic glory, hopefully brandishing your whip. Tell him that you are going to release him but he must understand that he must fully submit to your wishes. Ask him if he agrees to do so. If no, give him some more punishment. Tell him that he must address you as Mistress (or whatever you prefer of course). Unhook him and tell him to lick your pussy until you tell him to stop.

If he doesn't please you he will receive more punishment. When he has done so, tell him to go and stand back in the original place where he was secured and wait for you there. Remove his cock cage and squeeze his cock. Place the belt over the hook again so that he is standing there naked and vulnerable and tell him you are going to take some photos to send to his father. Take some photos on your phone and send them to someone you both know saying that you are training him. This is about public humiliation too so that when he sees that person, he won't know where to put himself and will be embarrassed about meeting them. Do it with someone he sees frequently but don't put his job in jeopardy please. Perhaps you could send it to one of your girlfriends so that every time you meet up you can both have a good laugh at his expense and make fun of his little penis. If he protests, ask him how he dare and give him some more punishment. Put the bag back on his head and leave him standing there, tied up and naked, for an hour or so.

When you return, tell him that you have received the ransom but before you release him, he has to service you to your satisfaction. Before releasing him, use a vibrator on his ass and tell him that that is the amount of pleasure you want to receive. Withdraw the vibrator before he comes. Bend over and tell him to take you from the back. Allow him to fondle and kiss your breasts and ask him to suck the nipples. Then stop him abruptly and tell him to get on with his job. When you have finished with him, release his wrists and tell him that he is free to leave but he knows you can come for him any time so always be aware that you can bring him back to do this all again.

Readers' Husband

Tell him that you have received a telephone call from a woman saying that she has spotted your husband at the supermarket and she is now having erotic dreams about him. She cannot stop thinking about him and imagining her hands all over him and being able to do what she wants with him. You said that you were not sure you could agree to that but she begged you and finally you agreed to take some erotic photos of him and send them to her. She said she would be willing to pay but you said that at this stage it would be all right for her to receive the photos for free.

If you changed your mind about sex in the future you might have to watch because he does belong to you and that includes his cock. Tell him that she was very grateful and you felt obliged to offer her this because she lives alone and is totally besotted with him. Tell him she asked you to describe his cock and what you get him to do to you and you told her that he was very good at licking pussy and made you come a lot. Tell him that you said that he liked to be spanked and that you have to keep him in control. She had asked if he would agree to the photographs and you told her that he had no choice because he had to do what you told him sexually.

She asked if she could be allowed to come round and take the photos of him herself but that she wouldn't want him to know it was her or he would recognize her when he saw her in the supermarket again. You had agreed that it would probably be all right but that she should wait to see if she wanted to take it further after seeing the photos you were going to send her. Tell him you found it erotic talking to her over the telephone because she was obviously becoming very aroused and you are sure that she had an orgasm because she was moaning and then screamed and that turned you on too. Say that you might consider a threesome or even a lesbian scenario when he has to watch. But not touch.

When he arrives home after work, tell him to strip off completely and you watch him. Lead him to the bathroom if he is not shaved and put him in the shower while you shave him. Lead him back to the bedroom. By this time he should be nice and erect so tell him that you have to have him inside of you before the session starts. Hopefully you should be nice and wet and ready for him by now but if you are not wet enough yet, rub some baby oil on his cock. Tell him to lie down on the bed and climb on top and ride him for all you are worth, satisfying yourself before the rest of the action begins. When you are finished stand up and get your camera ready. Start by taking some pics of his oily cock. If he has tried to come during the sex, stop him by slowing down. You could also slap his face to take his mind off his cock for a minute. You are in control and you want his cock nice and rigid for the photos. It would be great if you can manage to get a pic of his cock going into you.

Spend some time photographing him in various positions. Use your imagination but this could include him kissing your feet or sucking your toes, licking your pussy, sucking your tits. If you have a camera that you can put on a tripod, so much the better because then you can set it up to take pics of you sitting on his face or servicing you from the back.

You can also be inventive by getting him to kneel on all fours and sticking a dildo in his ass. Open the cheeks of his ass and get a good shot of his ass hole and put your finger in it while you massage his balls. Find the place that is very sensitive between his balls and asshole and stroke that too. Don't let him come because you want him to be erect for as long as possible and deferring climax will be torture for him.

After the session, tell him that you have got some fabulous shots and you are going to meet up with Carla tomorrow for coffee to pass them on and make sure she likes them. At the end of the next day tell him that you went to her house and ended up having sex with her because she got so excited and was so absolutely gorgeous you couldn't resist. Tell him that you ended up licking each other's pussies and sucking on each other's tits. You spanked her for being so naughty but you are going back for more because she was so juicy.

Tell him that she loved your photos and begged you to let her have a go on his cock and that you're considering it. You think you might like the idea of a threesome in fact. She is more than willing and asked if she could come and stay for a weekend and that she would agree to be their sex slave. Say that you told it would be better if both she and he were your sex slaves because you like to be in charge. Tell him she agreed to that and if he is a very good boy and does exactly what he is told, you will arrange it. Of course, he will be her sex slave as well and have to do exactly what you both instruct him to do.

You could show him the photos and tell him what she said to each one and that she started putting her hand in her pants at some point and rubbing herself but that you felt so turned on that you bent her over the table and knelt down and licked her pussy till she was screaming. Tell him that it is a new experience for you but one that you intend to repeat regularly and that she begged you to be her mistress and you agreed. Of course, this is role play but perhaps you will be both so turned on that you may want to turn it into the real thing.

Obviously, these are just a few ideas to set you on the path. I'm sure you have many more you want to live out. You will both find your own preferred level of pain and pleasure: you might not want any pain or you might want to experience real pain. It really is up to you.

Chapter Ten – Slice of Life

As much as I like to keep my life personal, there's so much I can teach my readers through my own experience back when I was still new to the FLR world, so I'm going to proceed to give you a gist of how I found out I was a dom, and how it all started for me. My first experience was not fantastic, but my second was what made me positive that I was meant for this life.

For as long as I can remember, I'd always been assertive and confident in my opinions. Growing up, through college, I'd thought my assertiveness was just a sign of confidence and a sense of self-worth. But that was until I met him. Now, for privacy reasons, I'm going to refer to him as Joshua.

It was sophomore year, and he had the prettiest face I'd ever seen. He usually sat in front of me, and I would notice how he would crane his neck toward me, pretending to borrow a pencil from his friend just to shoot me a glance. I was enchanted.

His hazel eyes glistened, and I felt tingling in my chest whenever he smiled at me, and his dimples sunk deeper into his face. I thought five years ago; I probably would have gone up to him, giggled like a dork, and waited until he asked me out. But I had grown up, and I was beginning to understand what I liked: how I liked my men and what I wanted to do with them.

I knew that through porn. When vanilla videos didn't cut it for me, and maledom videos made me uncomfortable, femdom films were this fascinating discovery that made me find my kinks. But I had never done anything like it, and it was only a theory of what I possibly liked.

And that was the thing. When I saw Joshua, I thought he was the perfect man to put the theory to the test. From the moment I laid my eyes on him, I knew he was going to be the first man I'd ever dominated.

He was nervous when I first approached him – nearly dropped his books. It turned me on how clumsy he had seemed. From a distance, he seemed to be the shy type who was going to continue being flustered until I set him straight. With my hand. Or maybe with a whip. I had already fantasized about it all before I said hello. I didn't know what he was into, but he seemed like the type who would let me do what I wanted to him.

And I wasn't wrong.

Of course, I was the one who asked him out. He was surprised by how confident I seemed – a remark which made me smile because it was almost like a code word for dominant. I thought it was a good sign that he could pick up on that. We walked to a local cafe, and I rushed to the door before he pulled it open for me. I didn't look behind me, but I knew the gesture made him smile. We sat down on a table for two, and I dismissed the waiter who came to our table too soon.

"We're still browsing the menu, thanks," I said, speaking on behalf of Joshua, as well.

I remember the way Joshua looked up at me with his toothy smile, his round cheeks pressing on his eyes as he squinted a little. My eyes were fixed on the menu, but I could see him looking at me. My legs were crossed, and my face was straight as I chewed my gum.

"You're kind of a badass," he commented in almost a murmur.

At this point, it felt like a cue for me to understand him more. I was intrigued, turned on, and almost star-struck.

"I bet you're equally as badass in bed," he continued with a smirk dawning on his face.

Until he said that.

Even though I'd been thinking of nothing but how I'd annihilate him in the bedroom, I didn't like how quickly he sexualized our encounter. I knew he was attracted to me from the way he subtly eyed me, scanning my body up and down and pausing at my bulging tits. But how quickly he had presumed that my approach was sexual turned me off. It was the kind of audacity that I never liked in a man. I liked them shy and reserved, leaving me the space to make the first move. But I didn't want to be picky, so I shrugged it off.

Fast-forward to when our food came, I was already bored out of my mind.

It had been fifteen minutes, and he wouldn't stop

talking about himself. He would sometimes let me comment, only to stop me and continue speaking his mind. The worst part was, he couldn't tell how cocky he was being. But aside from his unimpressive personality and juvenile intellect, that wasn't what bothered me. I felt like he had stolen control from me.

But he was a beginner, I was sure. I thought I could still train him. Clearly, he was sexually attracted to me strongly enough to go with the flow, and I still wanted to dominate him.

I asked for the check, and he didn't bother reaching for it. I didn't like that, either. It was almost like he was selectively submissive when it suited him, but still, I shrugged the second red flag off. I smiled at the waiter, my eyes following him until he left.

As soon as he did, I turned to Joshua and said, "So, are we doing this or what?"

He chuckled, almost choking on his own spit. "You mean, like," he paused, lowering his voice, "sex?"

"Clearly," I nonchalantly said, crossing my arms. "Since we both know why we're here, skipping class, we might as well just go for it."

"Fuck, that would be amazing," he said, his eyes growing wide like he had been waiting for me to say that.

Little did I know, this was not going to be a one night

stand, but a brief two-month relationship that felt a lot longer because Joshua, as I later found it, knew little about boundaries and personal space.

That afternoon, we walked back to my studio apartment. I kicked the door shut and smiled at him. He smiled back, blushing and glancing at the ground. I was really attracted to him at that moment. It was almost as though I only liked him when he revealed the shy and dorky side of him. I began undressing him, and he was about to undress me.

This was my chance to test it out.

"Don't touch me without permission," I ordered him with a straight face.

For a moment, he was confused. But as I continued to undo his belt, he smiled and understood where this was going.

"This is like, one of my biggest fantasies," he moaned as I pulled his pants down and began caressing his balls. "Fuck," he exclaimed in a whisper.

From the way it started out, I had thought this was going to go smoothly. But then he made those remarks that completely turned me off. As I stripped him naked, grabbed him by the chin, and looked him in the eye while I jerked him off, he said, "Yeah, you like that?" referring to his cock.

I wanted to roll my eyes. He wasn't doing this right. He

was too cocky, and it confused me more than anything. I was certainly attracted to him. I found myself smiling as I traced my fingers along the contours of his body, but the moment I looked him in the eye and saw how he smirked, it threw me off. He was a good looking man, but he knew that all too well, and it made it difficult for me to get in the mood.

But there I was. I had stripped a man naked and was leading him to my humble bedroom. When I turned around, I saw how he was checking out the place and nodding. He said he liked my lampshade and smiled. I hated that. He was opting out of our little power-play while we were in the midst of it. This guy clearly had no idea how to please a dominant woman.

I raised a finger to his lips. "Shut up," I said, trying to make it sound kinky as much as I could, but I really was annoyed with him.

He smirked again, seating himself on my bed as he licked his lips.

As I stood before him, glancing at his already hard cock, I kept thinking of how forced this felt. I didn't like how he treated it like a game. It wasn't a game to me; it was how sex should be. Surely, I knew that men were not really my servants, but I didn't like how Joshua reminded me of that by opting out of the dynamic every now and again.

I would have described him as someone who was too demanding, but I later discovered that he was needy, as well.

There he was, still on my bed. He looked up at me and pointed to his cock. "You can use teeth if you want. I like a little pain in that area."

You're not supposed to tell me that, Joshua, I thought to myself.

I was almost wet a couple of minutes ago, but now I was dry as a desert. I gave him a few spanks, and he smiled and giggled every time my hand landed on his round ass cheeks. I guess he really was submissive, but not the kind I liked. He didn't take it as seriously as I would have wanted him to. And I guess I also took him by surprise when I revealed I was a dom.

We didn't have sex that night. I didn't want to. He was disappointed, but he didn't say anything. He asked me to stay over, and I gave him no straight answer. He did anyway, and I later found myself caught in a relationship I never asked for. He noticed I wasn't happy with the way he presented himself to me, and he began to change.

But instead of changing into my type, he changed into this excessively needy idiot who would follow me around the apartment with nothing on but boxer briefs. He would sometimes purposely piss me off, thinking it would get him another spanking. Ironically, the last time he got on my nerves, it earned him a break-up. I asked him to leave, and he never stopped texting me since. He still does sometimes, and I cringe every time

I remember putting up with him.

Joshua made me question everything. I wondered whether the lifestyle I wanted was even real, or if it were just something idealistic that we only get to see in porn. I thought that perhaps my tendencies were best left in my fantasies, which I would maybe one day express through literature in an attempt to normalize FLR. Because, surely, if I could only see myself as a dom in any relationship, there must have been women out there who felt the same way. I just wasn't sure whether there would be enough men in the world who would mutually want such a relationship.

I wasn't exactly devastated, but I was definitely irked, and the feeling lingered for a few months until it slowly faded. It didn't dissipate, though. I always felt like there was something missing from my life, something that was never really going to be fulfilled because it was nothing but a fantasy inspired by adult films.

But that was until I met Brandon.

I didn't think much of him when I first met him. He was about the same height as me, but I always wore heels, so it felt like I towered over him whenever we talked. It was back in the corporate days when I worked next to him in a cubicle at a PR company. He would always try to find an excuse to speak to me, and I played along.

It was a few months until he seemed interested in me as more than just a colleague. I liked how he never flirted with me and only gave me the opportunity to initiate flirts. He was a funny guy and always made jokes about how I could easily destroy him if I wanted to. He was probably right, but I wasn't sure whether we thought of the same scenario.

I would catch him looking at me quite often, but he would always smile and look away. He rarely ever looked me in the eye for too long, especially while we made conversation. I liked how shy he was, and I eventually asked him out.

Brandon seemed surprised, but he never acted like too much of a dork. He was a shy gentleman who was as eloquent as he was kind. We were initially going to head to a nice cozy restaurant, but it was closed for renovations that night.

"Wanna get some corn dogs and take a walk?" he suggested, gesturing to the corn dog stand with his chin. He had his hands tucked into his pockets whenever he was around me. It was a little chilly at the time, but I knew that wasn't why he hid his hands.

I noticed how they shook a little whenever I was physically close to him. He was definitely attracted to me, and I was quickly growing to feel the same way.

I took the offer, and we went to get snacks. That day, I wore high-heeled boots, and whenever we were about to step down the sidewalk, he would link his arm with mine and help me down. I didn't need help, but I liked the gesture. Although he was shy, and I felt in control, he was still a gentleman that made sure I was comfortable.

It was always the little details that I paid attention to, like how he acted when we stopped by for ice-cream. The number of men that have said something along the lines of, "And perhaps a strawberry ice-cream cone for the lady?" made me think that men were just programmed to think that women liked everything pink and sweet. The only shade of pink I liked was a hand-print on a man's ass. And I guess Brandon, deep down, knew that.

He gave me the space to speak for myself and always listened when we conversed. Even though there was a back-and-forth, I still felt like I was the one leading it, and I didn't have to force it, either. That night, he walked me home and said goodnight. He stood there for a moment, almost slowly turning around to leave, hoping that it wouldn't be the end of it. I pulled him close and sucked a kiss out of his plump lips. I could feel him smiling on my lips. The kiss was slow and sensual, and he kept his hands to himself.

When I slowly pulled away, his face was flushed, and he kept combing his hair back with his fingers, flustered, and a little giggly.

"I think you just might be one of the most intimidating women I've ever met," he said, smiling. "I think it's my weakness."

That was it. I knew things would work out between us the moment he said that. He was the perfect blend of gentlemen and sub, and as much as I didn't want to rush things between us, I couldn't wait to have him in my bed.

Brandon was the one who taught me how FLR relationships should go. I'd previously thought that I had to make myself assertive in order to advertise myself as a dominant woman, but that was just the vulgar way to do it, and it attracted the wrong men. I later learned that you know a man is submissive when he gives you the space to make the first moves, while also very subtly expressing interest. They may initiate a conversation with you, but they rarely ever come forward with their feelings for you unless you allow them to. It all just comes naturally.

I had mistakenly thought that men had to be trained and informed of my ways, but I realized that I skipped quite a few essential steps. I was thinking with a sexual mindset, and that always ended up landing me creeps. There's more to an FLR than sex. Dominant women generally lead in the relationship, while also giving their partners the space to make decisions for themselves. This wasn't something that you sat down and announced to a man on a first date, but it was definitely something that you picked up on the more you socialized.

It was three dates later with Brandon until I invited him home. During these couple of weeks, we texted and face-timed. A lot. We talked about everything that we liked in more detail. That was when I realized that you should never surprise a man by the fact that you're a dominant woman. I thought I'd have to invite them over and surprise them with a whip, hoping they would be into that kind of thing. But that never turned out the way I wanted it to. Even when they were into it, it would all seem too forced, like it was an act on display.

That's why I brought it up to Brandon. We were exchanging provocative photos one day, and I straight up asked him if he would be interested in an FLR power-play in bed. He replied with, "You fucking bet," which was the fastest text he'd ever sent me, and it made me chuckle. He immediately confirmed that he was pursuing a mistress, but that he was also looking for a serious relationship. Just like me, Brandon was seeking a full-blown FLR. It seemed too good to be true, but there it was.

We agreed to meet that weekend, and we treated ourselves to steak and wine at a nearby restaurant. After he'd walked me home, I asked him if he wanted to stay over with me that night. His big brown eyes widened, and he immediately stuffed his hands in his pockets and swayed a little as he glanced at my front door. He nodded, then said yes.

I knew he was nervous. He knew exactly what was going to happen.

As I led him to the living room, I felt his eyes caressing me from behind, and he unsurprisingly looked away as soon as I turned around.

"You can sit down, you know," I said with a smile, looking up at him after he'd been standing over the sofa for a full minute, scanning my body with a shy smile.

He nodded and sat on the two-seater sofa with his hands on his lap. "So," he said, stifling a chuckle. "I'm sorry," he laughed. "I know you probably can't tell, but I'm just a little bit nervous."

I liked the way he sometimes mocked his own shyness, thinking it would turn me off. But it had the opposite effect on me.

"I like that you are," I replied, scooching closer to him.

He didn't look my way, but he smiled as he noticed I was almost close enough for my bare thighs to touch his.

Brandon's smile grew wider. "Do you like it when men are completely shaky leaves around you?"

I playfully rolled my eyes. "Sometimes. Let's just say I don't get along well with cocky men."

"I see," he nodded.

"Or generally dominant men," I clarified, reminding him of our conversation.

"That's comforting. I'm the complete opposite of all these qualities," he chuckled. "At least, that's what I recently realized, and it's probably why I haven't been dating as much," he said briskly, shaking his head as he spoke. He was still a little nervous, but he was getting used to being around me.

I put my arm on the backrest and played with his hair as he spoke. He paused for a moment, then continued, "But I feel more comfortable around you. I feel like women, in general, tend to expect me to get take care of everything for them," he paused, "Not that there's anything wrong with that, I'm just not that kind of guy, I guess."

I stifled a grimace. I remember how successful I felt at that moment like I had finally found the perfect guy for me. Still, I had no clue how rough I could be with him in bed, but even if I had to go easy on him, the man was worth it.

Brandon craned his neck toward me and glanced at my lips, squinting his eyes ever-so-slightly as if cueing for me to kiss him. I immediately leaned toward him, sucking on his bottom lip. He took in a deep breath and was smiling as I kissed him.

But he still kept his hands to himself.

I slid my hand to his lap, grabbing his hands and sliding them to my breasts. My eyes were closed, but I could feel him squirming a little. It was almost as though I could feel his heart beating. He was about to unbutton my blouse. U pulled back and slapped his hand.

"Did I grant you permission to do that?" I playfully snarled.

His chest was heaving. The more I got into character, the more it seemed to excite him.

"Sorry, mistress," he whispered. Finally, hearing someone call me that was like music to my ears.

Admittedly, I was becoming more impatient, and I immediately stripped him down. I hadn't even touched his cock yet, and he was rock hard. I loved how he knew that his hands had to be kept to himself unless I otherwise gave him permission to touch me.

It was kinky and sensual. It was the only sex I've ever had that felt real. I had been beginning to think that I was just not into sex since all it did was disappoint me. But with Brandon, with someone who allowed me to dominate him and actually enjoyed it, sex was captivating.

It was a night full of teasing, spanking, and fun punishments. He was also serious in his character, and he knew exactly what we were doing. That made it feel natural and spontaneous. It was exactly what I needed.

He stayed over that night, and we didn't stop talking since. We eventually dated, and power-play dominated (pun definitely intended) our everyday lives. He had quit his job at the PR company we worked at, and began working from home. He would let me know before I came home whether he was done with his projects. Whenever he had any tight deadlines, I would come back, order takeout, and we'd just watch some television before going to bed.

But on the nights both of us had the time, we would communicate via text beforehand, and it made it much easier and more natural for me to come home, not as Alexandra, but as Mistress. Sometimes, the power-play would start before I got home, too. I would order him to send me photos of himself in some poses, and he would abide. When I finally got home, that's when I'd decide whether I wanted to reward or punish him that night. He was always happy to get a face-sitting punishment, and his reward was either a blowjob or being allowed to penetrate me.

Our relationship was constantly evolving, and we always tried new things. Sometimes, he wouldn't like our new games, but he would go crazy about others. He was always open with me about what he was comfortable with; I was the same way. We never ventured with trying anything new in bed before discussing it beforehand.

If there was a formula for making this relationship successful, it was probably that period before we had sex, where we talked about everything we liked before giving it a try. Our first couple of times were magical, and the rest were full of experimentation and excitement. I thought I'd have to reveal the dominatrix that I am to men once we were in bed, but it turned out to be the least practical method I'd ever tried. I guess you could say I've learned that the hard way, and now I always talk to my partners before we decide to try out our roles, to see if both of us would be comfortable with it.

Conclusion

I hope you have enjoyed the book and that it has given you some ideas and helped you feel as if you are on an exciting journey to self-discovery and sexual fulfillment. It can feel lonely out there when you are just starting to explore the unknown territory and you feel like you're the only person on Earth that feels the way you do. This is amplified by the fact that dominant women are hard to find and men wishing to be dominated far outnumber them. But this goes to prove that it is a more common sexual proclivity than we might have initially thought.

I hope that you now feel optimistic about being a male submissive and that you have taken away new ideas of how to introduce this into your life. Now you know where to look for someone or how to introduce it to your current partner. Rarely does it exist in someone's life in entirety. In fact, I imagine that would be nigh on impossible but only you will know to what degree you can allow it into yours - or to what degree you wish to have it in your life.

I hope that the most important messages I have conveyed are that you are not alone, there is a growing number of men who are feeling more comfortable about admitting that they feel like this. You should also be confident about introducing the concept to an existing partner now too and fully appreciate how important discussion is within that relationship. It doesn't have to be the dominant factor in your life or your sex life and it's about finding a level that you are both comfortable and happy with. Your partner might only know how you feel if you tell her; she's not a mind reader. Even if the idea is totally taboo to her at first, give her time and show her ways that you can start with a light touch. Start treating her like a queen, buy her gifts, and surprise her with a sexy massage. Take your time to please her sexually and in day to day life. I guarantee that pretty soon she'll start appreciating all the extra attention and want to please you too.

All too often, people keep their thoughts and desires to themselves because they think that they're a bit off the wall or feel embarrassed or even ashamed of how they feel. If you can identify that this was you in the past, now you have the ammunition to get what you want for the future. Hopefully, this book has helped in your self-exploration and made you feel that it is quite normal to have these desires. In fact, I want to stress again, that as long as you are not hurting anyone, what you do in private is totally your own business and no one else's. Depriving yourself of things you want pleases no one so what is the point? You should live your life to the full and that should encompass your sex life too so don't be afraid to go out and get what you want.

I wish you well on your journey and hope you find fulfillment. In all areas of your life!

Before You Go

Please leave and honest Amazon review and don't forget to visit my site alexandramorris.com

Check out my other books:

Dominant Women

Erotic Hypnosis

Kink 101
Introduction to the submissive lifestyle

Dominant Women

The Dominant Women's and Submissive Men's Handbook for Amazing Relationships

information contained within this document, including, but
not limited to, —errors, omissions, or inaccuracies.

Introduction

The concept of dominance and submission is viewed as anathema in vanilla society. Most people don't understand how one can relish being submissive to another or give up that kind of control and trust another human being with their body like that. It is viewed as an outdated concept, and that's when the dominant is male and the submissive is female. The idea that a man might want to be the submissive is just inviting ridicule and disbelief.

Unfortunately, the benefits that bondage provides in a relationship with two consenting adults is often overlooked or simply not understood. So let us start from the beginning and define what dominance and submission mean. In the simplest terms, domination and submission refer to a power exchange between two consenting adults. The division between who is submissive and who is dominant is not limited by age, sex or gender. The level of domination and submission varies within relationships. In some it is limited solely to the bedroom, in others it carries on to other household dynamics. In very few of these relationships, it is a full lifestyle with the dominant making all decisions with total power control.

In what might be surprising to most people, the most common type of submission is male submission. This has been illustrated in erotic fiction and film, due to the appeal of thumbing a nose at the patriarchy. The domination of these males might be psychological or sexual in nature; being required to please their dominant before they are allowed to achieve arousal. In other cases, orgasm is denied until the dominant says they can come. This could be arbitrary or based upon certain behavior or completion of certain tasks.

Because it is traditional for males to dominate a relationship, flipping it and reversing it so that the female takes the Domme role can be sexually liberating and also very arousing. Since the act of sex usually involves inserting the phallus into the vagina, the male is often considered as the 'active' partner. The phallus actively penetrates the submissive vagina and so the latter is considered to be receptive. This leads to males fantasizing about male chastity in a bid to subvert this notion. It arouses them to relinquish control because they are expected to always be in control. To expound on this, it must be reiterated that the submissive does not submit by force. They willingly surrender all their power to the dominant. This can be a difficult concept to understand in that in a paradoxical way, the act of submitting and surrendering all power to the dominant is an act of dominance within your submission. The submissive always has a safe word, which they can use to immediately stop any activity they are tired of, are not in agreement with or would simply like to discontinue.

If the submissive feels unsafe, threatened, uncomfortable or scared by anything going on they invoke the safe word. It's their security blanket, which ensures that they will never be forced to do anything they don't want to or which is beyond their comfort levels or safety. This shows that the submissive is actually the one with all the power in the relationship because they have an emergency exit button that they can use at any time.

This book will look at the male submissive in a heterosexual relationship with a female Domme. As was mentioned earlier, this relationship might take place only in the bedroom or extend to everyday household activities. Male submission can also take place in a dungeon, with a professional Domme, using role play that is usually non-sexual in nature.

Research has shown that many high profile individuals faced with tough daily decisions at work where they are placed in high stakes dominant positions find sexual and psychological relief by being submissive in their relationships. The submissive role is stress relieving and liberating for them because they are constantly in charge of every aspect of their professional lives and give that control up in their sexual relationship. When they give up their power in this way, they not only relieve stress but it is also beneficial to them and their lifestyles.

Steve Jobs and Mark Zuckerberg have done interviews in which they both admit to wearing similar outfits on a daily basis in order to take away that one decision from the myriad ones they have to make every day. This helps them to focus on other things that matter more and helps them to do their jobs better.

In choosing submission, the man relinquishes his power in one way while still retaining it in all others. The use of a safe word enables them to have peace of mind as they willingly put their well being in someone else's hands. They are able to explore and bring to life their sexual fantasies and erotic thoughts without fear. Being able to do this is far from being helpless or powerless contrary to popular belief. This book will seek to debunk all the myths behind male submission and take a deep dive into what it means.

I have been inspired to write this book from my own experience because it so radically changed my life and my relationship with sex. I am a female in my early thirties whose sex life was what could always be described as satisfying, but after reading 50 Shades, something in my sexual psyche was awoken and I knew I must explore it further. The idea of sub/dom relationships always titillated my imagination and I was more than happy to try out a submissive role and found it erotic and stimulating. However, my partner confessed that he would like to try out adopting the role of submissive as well and I agreed that it was only fair that he get a chance to live out his fantasies too.

At first, it felt as if we were on totally unfamiliar ground and we were both feeling our way, uncertain of how we should progress exactly. I must confess that at first it did feel strange being the Domme because society very readily slots us all into our gender typical roles and we mature believing that we have found sexual gratification and often stop there without question.

However, for those of us who are more adventurous, we often find that, if we can release the inhibitions which are bred into us, we can discover a widely more satisfying experience altogether.

Our first efforts were tentative and unsure but we both soon gathered speed when we tasted how scintillating sub/dom sex could be. What drove us on was sheer passion and lust and we soon learned to overcome our inhibitions and enter into a rollercoaster journey of our erotic shared adventures together. We spoke about the limits we were both willing to endure and took pains to put each other at ease, building confidence in the other so that no actual fear was ever present. Needless to say, we trust each other implicitly, which I believe it paramount when setting out on this path, which, potentially, can present huge risks to its participants. We were explicit about how much pain we wanted to experience and the type of feelings we wanted to evoke. Some of our sex play was pure experimentation because I believe that sex should always involve the imagination and, for me, sex is as cerebral as it is physical.

I am lucky to have a partner who is as keen as I am to try out new things to keep our sex lives fresh and lively, and we talked about boundaries before we sprung anything on the other. Nevertheless, it did come as a bit of surprise when my partner said that he wanted to be the sub; it wasn't anything I'd considered previously. But because is always so obliging to my needs I was ready to give it a go if it meant it would enhance his experience. We were careful to agree on a safe word just as we had been when I'd been the submissive. I had thought it was probably going to be something we tried briefly and moved on from.

I have to confess that I did feel just slightly silly at first and a little self-conscious, even though we have always indulged each other's fantasies. As I relaxed though, I realized that was actually relishing the power that being the Domme gave me and I began to get into role and enjoy myself. I must have been convincing because it seemed that my partner was enjoying himself enormously too and rather than just trying it out and moving onto the next thing, we found that me adopting the Domme role became the fantasy of choice, which we seemed to indulge in increasingly until eventually it monopolized our sex lives completely.

I realized pretty quickly that I found it extremely liberating and that I enjoyed it more than I ever would have thought possible. It meant that I could be sure that sex was never hurried again. I could make sure I was completely satisfied in whichever way I felt like before agreeing to penetration or any other sexual gratification was allowed for my partner. He has a very demanding job and I think having an opportunity to relinquish the responsibility he has to wield constantly in a work environment was a complete relief for him. We normally keep sub/dom action to the bedroom, but he is catching on that if he is 'good' out of the bedroom he is more likely to earn sexual favors. His domestic prowess and involvement has certainly expanded and that makes me happier too. And, if I'm happier, then I'm more likely to be nicer to him too. He's more likely to come home bearing gifts now too, and it might be as simple as a bunch of flowers or a bottle of perfume – or even some type of sex toy. He enjoys seeing me happy and being the instigator of my happiness, which now very easily enters or sexual domain too. Our sex life, although it has always been good, has now reached new heights. I feel empowered and totally released from any past inhibitions.

We've started using costumes and sex toys more freely. He says that he finds my Domme persona hugely erotic and sexy and I like having complete control over him too. It does not diminish his masculinity at all for me and I feel cherished and adored by him. If anything, introducing this role play into our lives has improved our relationship on so many levels and I could never go back to vanilla sex. Our relationship has deepened and made us feel closer because it has introduced an intimacy between us that wasn't there before. It takes real trust between two people to give them license to hurt you. I think that we have achieved it and there will never be any looking back now. If you're nervous, start slowly and remember to keep talking to each other constantly about what you like and feel acceptable.

You'll never know if you never try it. Enjoy the exploration.

PART ONE: BEING A DOMINANT WOMAN

It might be difficult trying to remember when your sexuality was first awakened and how you felt. Similarly, it might be difficult remembering that first realization that you wanted to adopt the role of being a dominant woman, specifically sexually. Slowly, it dawns on you that vanilla sex might never be quite enough to satisfy you completely. Perhaps it was someone else who introduced you to this lifestyle and you realized how much more this extra dimension brought into your life. But when the relationship ended, new partners never had that same sexual proclivity and so you let it lie but thought you would never be fully satisfied again. So you resigned yourself to that fact and waited for someone else to come along and to light your fire. And then, you find someone who you are totally in love with and you settle down into marriage, never having discussed this desire because you feel embarrassed or a little afraid that he might think you're a freak.

Stop right there! If you are so in love with a guy that you are going to commit to him for life, then you need to discuss your innermost thoughts and make sure that you both trust each other with your lives and each other's body. If you commit to a life of vanilla sex without even exploring the options and keeping your mouth firmly shut, then you could potentially be signing up for a lifetime of boring and unfulfilling sex.

And committing your poor husband to be to a wife who he feels he can never satisfy sexually. So you need at least to discuss what turns you both on. Yes, of course he might be a bit stunned at first never suspecting his cute little angel could have anything quite so hot going through her mind. Or he might be so turned on by the idea that you go on to have the best sex you have ever had as a couple.

Whatever he feels, you should start by telling him how much it means to you and that you're not an expert by any stretch of the imagination. Like him, you are a novice and you would both be feeling your way along. You are about to open up to him and commit to each other in a way that is . My sex life had nearly always been satisfying but I will always be open to new ideas and like to try things at least once. Sub/dom was something I knew I wanted to continue to explore and the more repetition, the better. My first venture into this type of sex was as a sub and whilst I enjoyed this, I knew that I might probably be happier in the role of the Domme. When I first suggested that I wanted to be spanked by my partner, he readily agreed and seemed to enter into it wholeheartedly.

Little by little, we introduced more sub/dom sex play into our sex lives and spiced things up so much that we both soon realized that we might want to go further. I was only slightly surprised when my partner suggested that he might enjoy being spanked by me and even though I felt a little self-conscious to begin with, I soon became aware of how much I was enjoying myself.

From there I could quite easily progress onto demanding sexual acts be performed on me such as oral sex and I could make it last for as long as I wanted to without feeling pressurized by thinking he might not want to do it for long. We spoke about our feelings openly and he told me how much he enjoyed satisfying me and being told what to do by me for me.

We both felt as if our sex lives had opened up and expanded into unknown, naughty but nice territory. I found erogenous zones on his body that he had never asked me to touch before. And I guided him to new ones on me. We progressed to canes and belts, but I took care to monitor the strength I used until I knew exactly how much pressure to exert. We both felt much more sexually adventurous and daring and our conversation about sex became more uninhibited and freer. We were not afraid or embarrassed to discuss anything with the other, which bonded us closer than we had ever felt before and welded our sexual partnership together with trust.

We had been seeing each other for around two years when, out of the blue, he was offered a job that was too good to refuse. To cut a long story short, and after much angst and discussion, we decided that he should go alone. I work in a high-powered industry too and love my job. We said that if our relationship were strong enough, then we would come back together in the future. When he went, he left a big hole in my life, emotionally and sexually, and I realized that when I was ready to look for a sexual relationship with someone else, it might involve going back to basics with a new partner. Alternatively, I knew that there are clubs and support groups where you can find like-minded people, or even on-line, which can make it easier establishing a new partnership. All hope was not lost, and I began to explore my options.

For some, it might feel a little seedy when visiting clubs where sex, and what most still consider to be *kinky* sex, is the prime motivation for visiting but if you can take it in the spirit of fun then it becomes much easier to loosen up and be open with others. I toyed with this idea and decided to give it a go. I persuaded an open-minded female friend to come with me – I wasn't brave enough to go alone at this stage – and, at first, we just looked on it as a recce. We were just testing the water and would see what turned up, if anything. I wasn't holding out much hope. My friend openly admits that she is more comfortable with a sub role and this type of relationship is more prevalent. She met someone on our first visit, and they went onto continue seeing each other for over a year.

For me, on the other hand, it was more difficult. I don't think that I was unnecessarily choosy, but I wanted to make sure that it was someone who turned me on and with whom I had other things in common. Some people feel differently to me and for them it's all about the sexual relationship; in fact, it can be almost anonymous. But I had not long come from a stable, loving and trusting relationship and I felt that anything less would not be enough, it would simply be a compromise. For that reason, I decided to take my time and hoped I would recognize the real thing when he appeared. There were a few dalliances, but no-one seemed to fit the bill and I recognized that they would never be anything more than ships that pass in the night but still enjoyable and mostly worthwhile experiences. Whilst some managed to add to my experience, I did find that not all preferences matched mine either. The trick is to take it slowly and see what suits what people in the relationship, literally to feel your way. Taking it slowly also fosters extra safety measures and excellent and clear communication is a must. We're all so different and our sexual preferences, just like any other preference, will vary from person to person. Be clear about what you want and be honest with the other person about whether you are willing to fulfill their desires too. Be as explicit as you can and agree guidelines so that there are no misunderstandings.

Start Slowly

You might experience feelings of guilt to start with, and this is quite understandable because all through your life you have been indoctrinated that your place in a male dominated society is to serve men. This might be especially true if you were raised in a religious home where anything outside the dictates of what is regarded as vanilla sex is denigrated as being taboo. Your guilt is just an indication of how well and how long women have been suppressed under male dominance.

However, there are two sides to this coin and as society changes around us because of the introduction of technology and its rapid pace, man's role within it changes too. Whereas men might have expected to have manual jobs and a clearly defined role that was physical and masterful, the need for such jobs is quickly disappearing. He finds himself floundering in a world where he is beginning to feel superfluous to requirements. He becomes unsure of his identity and who he really is. However, he might have been raised in a household where his father was the patriarch and anything that he could not understand was ridiculed or abhorred. So the man you meet now has been very well trained to stay within those parameters. To step outside of them would cause him immense guilt too. And he is used to seeing his mother playing the little woman at home. Add to this that he might be a university graduate who has progressed into a high-powered job where he is expected to take decisions which might even affect others' lives on a daily basis. He is constantly stressed but gets on with the job at hand because that is what is expected of him. Since he was born, not only has his family drilled into him that he must be a man and provide for his family, but films and media have contrived to push this fact home to him. But now everything around him is changing and he is left in a confused state of flux.

When we look at it like this, men are having just as hard a time as women in adapting to the new dictates and requirements of a civilization which is driven by technology and roles in general are changing out of recognition to those of just a few decades ago. Alongside that, sex is becoming more visible and vocal. People are beginning to break out of the closet and stand up for what they really want and be who they feel they are, instead of pretending to fit the standard one size fits all. Try and see yourself as a suffragette for women's rights and you are participating in actions that will rid women of any guilt and shame that may have been inculcated within them to keep them in their place. Communication with your partner is the key. You should both be there to help and support the other one on their journey. Do not try and launch into a fully blown S&D relationship. Take your time and get to know what you and your partner enjoy. Liken it to learning to drive. You would not expect to get into the driver's seat and know immediately how to drive without making any mistakes along the way. It is a process that has to be learned like any other and the more information you can gather, the quicker the process is made and the more confident you will both become.

Your partner may feel much more comfortable if your dominance is combined seamlessly with romance. Ask him to make you feel like a lady again. Tell him you want him to write you love letters or poetry and recite them to you. Tell him you want to recapture the romance you used to feel. If your partner has expressed the sentiment that he will never be able to let you whip him, then you must find another route to your destination. It might take longer to arrive than you wanted it to but if you apply the right attention it will be well worth the wait. Even the greatest of studs who consider themselves sexual champions can be shocked when female dominance is first suggested to them. Instead, this might suggest that rather than being the open-minded liberal they thought themselves to be, they are encased within their own masculinity – or their idea of what a masculine man should be. Any thought of relinquishing this could fill them with a horror of their abrupt emasculation.

Imagine a male dominant having the roles reversed. How would he be likely to approach the subject of domination of his partner? Typically, he would not ask for permission or say that he would like it to be discussed before entering into the action. At best, he might ask his partner what she likes sexually, but quite often it is taken as read that the woman is enjoying whatever a confident dominant submits her to. In fact, even when she asks him to stop – or even begs him to – he may still assume that this is still part of the game and continue. She may well have to scream 'rape' before he puts the brakes on and comes to realize that she actually means what she says.

If you find yourself in a sexual relationship with a man like this, it may be what you prefer. However, if you want to be able to turn the tables, you have many tricks up your sleeve at your disposal. Your arsenal is the most powerful of all the sex tools. You may have to be more persuasive, but there is always a way to get a man to do as you wish. If he tries to insist on being the dominant partner, you must show him quite firmly that you are not agreeable to it. If he tries to force you, then delay enjoyment for him. Set him tasks to perform like cooking a meal for you. When he does something that pleases you, reward him. This might just be by giving him a very long sexy kiss. Dress for the part and laugh at the same time, don't be put off your stride if he tries to pull you towards him and take over your plans. Or you might just stroke his penis through his pants. Or you could put both hands inside his pants and squeeze his ass cheeks while you're kissing him. Try being rough in bed and you take the lead. Pull his hair while you are having sex. Initiate sex when you feel like it, not when he does, and deny him sex when he does. Brush up on where his erogenous zones are and try them all out to establish which is the most powerful to get his engine running.

Flirt with him. Flirting is such a potent aphrodisiac. Tell him what you want him to do to you. Have phone sex with him. Ring him at work and whisper very dirty things into his ear, especially when you can be sure that someone else is near to him and might overhear you speaking on his phone.

Buy him presents such as a cock ring and you put it on him. Buy him a chastity belt and insist he wears it. In bed, make sure you climb on top of him so that you can regulate the sex. When he is about to climax, climb off and say, *"Not yet big boy. I'm not ready. You will have to please me a lot more than that."* And then sit on his face and tell him to lick your pussy because it's getting far too wet. You regulate the timing until you make it excruciating for him and he begs you to let him come. Don't let him until you are ready. Make it the best night he has ever had. Make him bend over and try fucking him, maybe with a strap-on dildo you have bought or your own vibrator. Or perhaps with a finger at this stage.

When you have serviced him, tell him to get up and get you a glass of wine or cup of coffee. Say that you are only having a rest and you need more of him so that he can't go to sleep just yet. Ask him to rub your whole body down with oil and then offer your breast for him to suck. While he's doing that, keep telling him that he's a good boy and that he's doing a good job. He's really turning you on. Now tell him to rub your clitoris just the way you like it. There is only him that does it right because he's so good. He gives you it just the way you like it. Keep giving him a little bit at a time. Get on all fours and tell him to fuck you from the back. The way that you're introducing your dominance is very subtle. You're asking him to do things for you but then praising him and telling him that he's the stud. Intersperse this with normal requests such as could he get your phone for you because you can hardly walk after the seeing-to he's just given you. If he tries to mount you without being instructed to do so, tell him to get off you because you're in charge tonight and you want to save some for him so that you can go on for longer and give him what he deserves. If he tries to spank you, slap him and tell him that is not allowed. Bit by bit, you are taking his power away from him and before he knows it, he will be eating out of your hand.

Remember always to assume the position on top during sex until he gets used to the idea that you are in charge.

As he becomes more and more used to the things you want to introduce, start bringing more things into it: gags, butt plugs, blindfold and hand-cuffs. Keep telling him that he is really turning you on and that you can't get enough of him. If he carries on you are going to suck his cock like he's never had it sucked before. When you do that, put a finger up his ass and with a finger on your other hand, gently squeeze his balls and stroke the part between his balls and his anus. This should turn him on so much that he is putty in your hands.

Keep the impetus going by reminding him the next morning how much you enjoyed yourself and then ask him to bring you breakfast in bed because you are so exhausted and you have to gather your strength so that you will be able to repeat it. Inch by inch, introduce him to new experiences and these should be interspersed with tasks you wish to delegate to him. If you haven't been able to get him to do the garden, for instance, promise him a night to remember if he makes a start on it immediately. Of course, you are using sex to get what you want. But why wouldn't you? You are both getting what you want and you not only get the house looking good, but you get to live out your fantasy of being a female dominant. If you're clever, he won't even be aware you're doing it. He will be very grateful for the marvelous sex life he's been gifted with.

Greet him when he returns from work wearing nothing but stockings, high heels, and a hat. Tell him you want him now and instruct him to strip off completely and fuck you over the kitchen table. Then tell him to order food and open wine and you lounge around on the sofa telling him to hurry up and come and satisfy you quick. I doubt that he'll refuse.

So from being in a partnership with a macho dominant man who you loved in all other respects, he is quickly growing into the completely ideal man you have been seeking all your life. You could also introduce your man to female dominant literature and films. How would he like to have a zany, erotic and exotic night out? Tell him that you have to dress up in fancy dress and that you are going to meet lots of wild and colorful people. Be upbeat and enthusiastic about it. After visiting such a place, he might find that he's had such an excellent time that he wants to go back.

Another way of playing out your dominance with a hitherto dominant man is to suggest cuckolding. Quite often this turns on a man who perceives himself as being macho. He enjoys seeing other men having a good time with his partner and being able to be present makes him feel complicit in the naughtiness. He might think because it is not within the realms of what is considered normal by society at large, that he is being naughty too. So this takes us back to when he was little again and is still a form of male submission. The woman is being fucked by another man right in front of him and he is actually giving his consent for her to do so. Who is in charge of the situation?

Equally, most men seem to be turned on by seeing two women together. If you are bisexual or even you could quite easily convince your partner to comply with our wishes that you have sex with other women as long as you allow him to watch. He is not allowed to have sex with her, and he might not be allowed to watch you either having sex with a man or another woman. However, he will be incredibly excited by the prospect of you telling him exactly what happened afterward and promises him that he is promised the night of his life afterwards because the whole experience makes you feel so horny. He should lap it up and be eating out of your hand – or pussy – on command before you know it.

There are so many degrees and differences within S&D, so many variations of what it constitutes, so much for you to explore. So it is going to take a lot of discussion between the two of you and a lot of experimentation. The frequency and intensity is something that you will not know when you first start. In fact, you might not even know where or how to start. The first place perhaps to explore is through the Internet, magazines, movies, and books. At the end of your research, you might decide that you want to start off softly, but then after doing the same thing repeatedly you want to go a little deeper and be more daring and adventurous. Like anything else, if you do something over and over without changing it at all, it is likely to become boring and predictable, so try to be open-minded to keep things fresh and exciting.

You could start by buying some sexy underwear. Images of female dommes are prevalent and easily obtained all over the Internet but no doubt you or your partner may have something in mind already. If you feel embarrassed about buying these in person, have a look for something online so that it can be sent to you discreetly. Even wearing sexy underwear under your work clothes can give your sex life a new lease. You don't have to build the dungeon in your basement immediately, as soon as you get agreement from your partner to try S&D out. Don't splash out on a load of expensive equipment to start with. You might find you've shelled out a month's salary on stuff you're never likely to use again. Use your imagination in as many areas that will improve your sex life as you can. Improvise with equipment. No one says you have to have metal handcuffs and a whip, especially not to begin with. What's wrong with a scarf and your hand, or even a belt if you both agree to it?

No doubt you are both going to feel self-conscious at first but once you start to grow in confidence this will disappear and you will be more ready to experiment with other things. Some couples might agree to visit a club and there are many around, some dedicated to male domination. Have a look and research what's near you. If you have to travel a good distance, make it a special event. If you do, try and see it for what it is: fun. You don't have to join in with anything but dress up and get in the spirit or otherwise you're liable to stand out like a sore thumb and look like tourists. Even observing others or talking to more experienced people will give you invaluable lessons that you might not be able to learn elsewhere. It will also make you identify with a group and help to satisfy those feelings that may be lurking in the recesses of your mind that you are abnormal. Don't take your parents with you in your head or this might never work. On the other hand, there's nothing wrong with feeling naughty. Sex can be naughty but nice.

At this stage, it is more about communication with your partner. Talk about what he would like to try out to persuade him that it might be well worth a try on some level. You can work out what to move onto as you go along. Ask him about what turns him on. What are his fetishes? Encourage him to open up to you. What you are aiming for is equality in the relationship, one that is mutually satisfying so you tell him what you would like to try too. But don't try and rush things too quickly. Slowly, slowly catchy monkey.

If you do feel embarrassed at first, then try and go with the flow. Don't take any negative comments from your partner personally. If he asks you to do something differently, do not take it as a criticism but try and see this as part of the learning curve. If he puts you off, by commenting about something negatively while you are actually doing it, forbid him to speak during the session. Something like that could knock any confidence you were carefully building up right out of you. Confidence is of paramount importance when assuming the role of a Domme. If you don't feel it at first, fake it. You have to be credible for the persona to be effective so you must show him that you are the one in charge. Dressing for the part can help, both to get you to feel in character and it speaks volumes about the role you are adopting. Don't forget to use the posture and body language too. Feel the part and after a short time, it will begin to feel natural.

However, this is not to say that you shouldn't discuss it afterward. You want to learn from your experience and make them as pleasurable as you can for each other. Of course, you will make mistakes. We all do, and you would be unnatural if you both did everything perfectly at first – either that, or very low in expectations. It is a game and is to be enjoyed. You both make your own rules because it is your own personal game. You are devising it and making it up as you go along. Share the experience as fully as you can. It should be fun and if one of you is not enjoying it, you need to discuss openly why not and decide what you can do about it to ensure that both of you enjoy it in future.

However, do not be persuaded to do something which you do not wish to do, however heartfelt his pleas. If you start going against your natural instincts you are being controlled and manipulated, exactly the opposite to what you are hoping to achieve. Be steadfast. If you discuss it and you still feel the same at the end of the discussion, then say so and state your reasons why. And stick to your guns.

When you ask him questions or ask him to describe what he likes, don't just hear it but actively listen. If you do this, it should become a fuller and more comprehensive conversation and help you to give him exactly what he wants. If he does become overly critical of you during the session, then remind him that he is there to please you. Of course, this would not apply if you are crossing the thresholds that you should have agreed before commencing the threshold. He is your servant and you must tell him that he is now going to be punished for his words. Make it part of the session. Try and force yourself to be dominant at first because you will grow into the person you are wishing to be if you act if out regularly.

Try and find a support group. This is not just for when you are starting out but can be seen as an ongoing group identity and offer support for whenever you flounder. You also get the chance to share what you've learned so far too with other women who might need the support just as much as you once did. Sometimes, it can help to talk to others who are in the same position as you. You can offer each other moral support and suggest solutions to any problems they are having but which you have managed to overcome. If you can't find any in your area, look for one online or start your own. Members of a peer group can suggest new things to try that have been successful for them so that it can help you to introduce new things that you might not have thought of or come across otherwise yourself. When you're feeling abnormal, peer group members can talk you through it and assure and convince you that whatever you choose to do within a loving relationship is perfectly acceptable. They are like any other friends you have but they add another dimension that your friends who are not part of an S&D relationship might not understand or be able to offer support around.

What if you are inexperienced when it comes to S&D and have been married or in a stable relationship when your partner suggests that he would like to try out this lifestyle? What should you do? Well, first of all, try not to be shocked at his proposal. He may have suppressed his longing for some time and be nervous or even afraid of suggesting such a thing to you for fear that you might see him differently or reject him. But he is still the same person who you loved before he told you of his desires. In fact, you should feel honored that he has finally found the courage to share his innermost desires. Ask him to tell you more about it and ask for more information on the subject. He may have had time to find out a lot of information while he has fought his inclinations and tried his best to suppress them. Be aware that he could have gone and paid for a professional domme to fulfill his fantasies but instead, he has chosen to confide in you because he loves you. You are his queen and he wants to make your love life more satisfying for both of you.

If you do feel disgust or shock, try and question why you do so. Are your reactions perhaps more to do with your own relationship with sex rather than his? Try and be open-minded and receiving. Don't push him away. Together you have found out that you can overcome most obstacles in your path or at least find a way around them. There is no reason why this one should be any different and you might discover that it introduces something into your life that could be so wonderfully exhilarating and new. Be very honest and open about your thoughts. Perhaps he can help to dismiss any doubts you may feel, perhaps not, but you will never know unless you try. Respect him for his honesty and his strength. If you tell him that he should be ashamed at this stage, there might be no way of bridging the gap that you create by your harsh words about something which is very personal to him and part of who he is. It's natural that you should be filled with all kinds of unusual and maybe unwanted emotions when your husband/partner reveals his proposals. But rest assured, he is not a pervert or a freak or even abnormal, whatever your instincts guide your thoughts towards.

If you love each other, there is always room for negotiation to reach a compromise or agreement where both members of the partnership can be happy and flourish. But be warned, once you have enjoyed sex as a dominant woman or generally been dominant in your everyday lifestyle, it is always going to be difficult for you to revert to a life without it. Sex might be good in the future without your dominance being a feature of it, but it will always seem like flat Champagne, however good it gets.

Personally, I prefer serious relationships where trust and love build up over time. I'm not saying that this is the only sort of relationship within which I've had sex, but I find I don't feel confident enough to express my dominant side with someone I don't know well. I know that some women to prefer it with partners who they do not know as well as they might and that this can add a titillating and exciting dimension to the S&D experience. It is a personal thing, and this is only something, which you can decide is the preferred avenue for you to follow. I feel personally safer and freer to be myself within a committed and close relationship. For me, it's just another element of expressing how much I trust my partner and a way that he can reciprocate his total trust in me. When I see how much he wants to please me in every way, it is clear evidence of his devotion to me. He knows that he will get exactly what he wants if he takes the time to please me too instead of solely considering his own needs. It's a way of keeping that interest alive instead of sex becoming mechanical and predictable. I like to explore everything that occurs to me and my partner. It keeps our sex life refreshing and exciting. I never want to say that I suffer boring sex. And I don't.

Different Ways of Being a Domme

Being in an S&D relationship is not all about sex exclusively. Men want to adopt the lifestyle in all sorts of degrees, and this could incorporate financially, domestically, completely. Again, it's about negotiation and about what you both feel comfortable with but there are ways of subtly introducing S&D if you are not ready to introduce it in its entirety or neither of you wish to do so.

When this is first introduced to a woman by her partner, the woman often wonders where it has come from. Previously, she might have regarded her relationship with her partner to be perfectly acceptable and she was always satisfied with her sex life and her married life in general. But now her partner wants to introduce this new facet into their lives, and she may be nervous about having the dynamics of their relationship tossed around and disturbed for potential destruction. What she must consider is that her partner has perhaps struggled with the concept for a long time and it has taken a lot of courage to introduce the idea to her.

Communication might open up to reveal that he is more interested in being controlled in other ways than sex. But it is likely that this proclivity probably stems from the relationship he developed with his mother or some other authority figure in his formative years. All he wanted to do then was to please that important woman who nurtured him and took care of him and disciplined him when he needed it. Hopefully, she was firm but fair. He felt cared for and loved and that has sunken deep into his psyche and is an essential part of who he has become. It is only natural then that he would like to recreate this feeling with another significant woman in his life: you. Do not take his proclamations lightly. If you are shocked or alarmed, do your best to hide it. The very worst thing you can do is make him feel abnormal so that he shrinks back into himself and decides to satisfy his needs elsewhere.

Holding the power in a relationship might not involve all black leather and bondage. It can be much more subtle than that and it is much easier to introduce if this is the case. When you are in bed, ask him to do something for you and if he is reluctant to do so or even refuses, stroke his penis, nibble his ear or perform whatever really turns him on. It doesn't have to be about performing actions that you might consider irregular or outlandish. This is more about timing and reminding him of how much pleasure you can give him if he treats you right. If you are confident about who you are and the sexual being that you are, this is an easy step to being able to get him to do whatever you want. Some women give their gift away far too easily and cannot understand why games must be played. However, if you don't value the marvelous gift you can bestow upon the chosen ones, why should anyone else value it? You have already proven to them that they don't have to prove themselves to you, that sex with you is on tap whenever they want it. Being permitted to have sex with you is like brandishing the metaphorical whip and it is surprisingly easy how men can quite rapidly change their minds with a bit of oral sex. But in order to receive, they must give, and you should make them work for it.

Since time immemorial, women have had the power to rule the world. And their partner. All you have to do is to grow into your power and make sure that you feel like the sex goddess you want him to see you as. Walk around as if you own the world and notice if men turn to look at you when you enter a room. Women do not have to be incredibly beautiful to attract attention; it is all about confidence. So start building it. And as your confidence grows, so will your partner's wish to fulfill your desires and receive favors from you. Sexual favors are not a joke, but it is something that has been portrayed as one as women's emancipation grows in society. Wanting equality can be a two-edged sword because it can so easily change the dynamics in the bedroom as well as the boardroom. You want your partner to see you as the most desirable woman in the world so act like one and the feeling will become real.

Try and discuss all aspects of being dominant to his submissive. How far does he wish to adopt this lifestyle? As you can see from above it doesn't have to take large leaps away from your normal sex lives. It can just be a redress of balance within the partnership. There are so many different ways you can incorporate female dominance and you might find that one runs on quite naturally from quite a tame start and develop into eye-popping raunchiness. You see it as a way to improve your life, which may or may not include domination. Your partner sees it as a way to get more sex and to fulfill his fantasies. Everyone's a winner, one way or another.

Various other suggestions that he might run past you might include one or more of the following:

Financial

This is often referred to as Findom and is more or less self-explanatory. Whether or not one or both of the couple works, the woman is in charge of the financial side of the household. Get his name taken off the joint bank account. Anything he earns must go into your bank account. This might involve her taking complete control of all finances and giving the man an allowance on which to manage despite him being the largest earner. Once you have complete financial control everything else should fall into place nicely. You can have a power of attorney so that you are allowed to sign for anything in place of your partner. You will pay all the bills from their joint income and make all financial decisions. You will decide how much you as a couple can spend on a social life, clothes, holidays and household bills.

Your partner receives an allowance decided upon by you, either weekly or monthly, but he must make a report to you of what he is spending his allowance on. Make him provide receipts and a weekly spreadsheet or list of expenditure. For anything he needs outside of his allowance he must make a special request to you and it is ultimately your decision whether or not he gets it.

Despite this sounding something he might wish to avoid at all costs, it does have benefits for both people in a partnership. At least when only one person is in charge of finances, there can be no misunderstanding about who has paid the bills or what is going out of the bank account. So there are no nasty surprises to be had because the female plans it all out. Be aware though, should anything go wrong, the blame comes to lie firmly at your door so don't see this as a license to spend, spend, spend on every frippery you see.

It also allows the male to step back and relinquish control, which he might welcome; especially should he have a stressful job. He might be involved in number crunching all day, every day at work, so the last thing he wants to do is come home and manage the household too. By giving his partner control, he is satisfying a basic need of being cared for and cherished. Conversely, if you take control of the finances, it can be an extra burden for you to stress you out. Weigh this one up carefully before you try and wrestle control because it can be more trouble than it's worth in the long run to have to balance the books constantly, especially if money is tighter than you would wish.

Household Chores

Is there anybody out there who genuinely enjoys domestic chores? Cleaning the toilet? Washing the dishes? The endless vacuuming of carpets or mopping? By doing the household chores, your partner is showing you how much he cares for you and this might explain why so many dominant women enjoy and embrace such a lifestyle. Give him lots of encouragement and praise and cuddle him or promise him something sexy you are sure he will enjoy.

You might choose to incorporate this part of your dominant role into your S&D lifestyle in a big way and use it to humiliate him, thereby exploiting his submissive desires to the full. And how often, when your house needs cleaning, do others blame the woman for being a dirty slut? They might profess to be modern thinkers, but it is when outmoded views like this escape them, you realize at once how deeply entrenched our society believes that the woman's place is in the kitchen. Well actually, it's not. But it can be in the bedroom sometimes.

When the S&D role play is more pronounced in the relationship, to encourage him to take a more active role in the housework, for instance, and in your strict dominant role, you might instruct him, in your most bitchy voice, to brush the toilet floor using a toothbrush because he seems to be neglecting the corners. Insist that he continues to clean it until it is up to your satisfaction. You could insist that he carries out household chores wearing only an apron – provided he can't be seen too easily by the neighbors through the windows! Quite often, because women have adopted the domestic role from the start of the relationship, she has grown used to doing things in her own inimitable style and her partner's efforts might not be quite up to par as far as she is concerned. Agreeing to incorporate the domestic side because of his submissive nature answers both of your needs perfectly. He gets to exploit his submissive side and you get the housework done to your satisfaction. It's not good for him to cut corners. If he is going to go along with this agreement, make him do a good job otherwise what's the point of it. He might be getting something from it – but it's in his own head only – and what's in it for you. Use your head - as well as other bits of you to get the best out of him.

Childcare

If you have children, you already know how stressful this can be, especially if you work as well. Running them to school each day in peak hour traffic is no picnic and studies have shown that a mother's heart rate can rise significantly during this journey. Add to that, that the kids are screaming for whatever they want at the moment and you have a pile of ironing to do after work. That is after you have called in at the supermarket to pick up whatever you're having for dinner and having to race around it at a breakneck speed so that you are there to pick up the kids in time again. How much easier would it be if you have a househusband at home who can relieve you of all this pressure? Even if he still works, or maybe works from home, he can still relieve you of the most onerous tasks while you have a relatively easy day at work, socializing with workmates and enjoying what you do.

Feeling challenged intellectually is something that stay at home moms can miss and don't realize how much their lives are going to change by having children. However, because of societal changes precipitated by technology and women's rise in status, their traditional roles are evolving into something totally different to those their mothers and grandmothers might have experienced. A domestic role reversal might be truly appreciated by the man of the family who welcomes a break from what he has been trained to comply with from birth. Being at home with the children releases him to explore his feminine, softer side and can be beneficial for the children. They learn to adapt to the new world that is evolving around them and trains them to live comfortably and easily within it. They also benefit from having a male role model feature prominently in their lives, and this is especially true of a man who is unafraid of showing his softer, feminine side. He also gains by getting to know his children better and being a much stronger influence in their upbringing and the shaping of their characters.

Different Measures of Success

Everyone is different, as you will soon discover when you start the journey of BDSM. Your partner may well be very different to anyone else you might have met or shared such a relationship within the past. What you are both exploring is how to meet in the middle and share common experiences from which you both benefit. Why would you protest against your partner wanting to please you? It is just a question of working out how that is best achieved. He might want to only take parts out of the lifestyle, which are not highly sexual. If he does wish to participate in sexual role-playing, he may be selective in what he wishes to practice and you both have to communicate your needs to the other to discover what they want. It is always about mutual satisfaction.

First, establish what you ideally would want and then use that as your starting point. It will be highly unlikely if your partner agrees willingly and gladly to all of your suggestions immediately and without protest. If he is completely taken aback by what you are suggesting, then try to convey how important it is to you and how you could introduce diluted forms of it. While he might be very adamant that he does not want to be involved in sexual domination, he might be quite willing for you to make all the major household decisions or those involving the children. This might be a good time to show him how much of a sexy woman you can be and where sexual favors could be very neatly introduced. With just a little persuasion, say stroking his penis, and giving him wet and penetrative kisses, he could easily change his mind or at least warm to the idea. Eventually, you might get him to the stage where he knows to battle against you is futile.

You may both lead a very active social life. You might make it a rule that he must always consent you when he is going out with anyone but you and give you plenty of warning when he intends to. Never be satisfied with a last-minute call that he has decided to stop off for drinks with friends at the expense of wasting the wonderful dinner you might have prepared for him. It is just common courtesy and you should never be afraid of demanding that.

Whatever shape or form your relationship takes, it should be developed within a safe and caring relationship. Do you, for instance, want to be treated like his queen and worshipped? This might involve running you a nice relaxing bubble bath and washing your hair, after which he could gently towel you down and blow-dry your hair. Get him to do your nails while he's about it. So far, nothing overtly sexual has occurred, but then if you go onto have sex afterward, you might command him to give you a massage followed by shaving your pubes and then licking your pussy until you have an orgasm. When you're entirely satisfied and relaxed you can perhaps allow him to have sex with you but you choose the position and he has to obey. You might even allow him to come if you are feeling generous. Nothing unusual or untoward has happened. At least nothing you or most other people would consider outside the realms of a normal sexual relationship. He may or may not realize that you have already introduced an element of S&D into your relationship and that he didn't find it too unpalatable; he might even have enjoyed it immensely.

He doesn't have to be a total pushover either. You don't want him to end up as a total wimp do you? So again, careful discussion must be allowed to take place. Let him have his say. He might not want it public that he is your sex slave every weekend and that he is subjected to being whipped or having butt plugs inserted. Or that you insist he wears women's underwear to work everyday under his very formal business suits. Conversely, he might relish the fact that you are telling all your girlfriends what you get up to in private, especially if you can tell him truthfully that they are now all working on their partners to get the same treatment. When he sees them eying him up knowingly and admiringly, hopefully that is going to make him feel good and make him even more willing to cooperate.

Blend the treatment that you dole out so that even though you might be telling him he has a small penis, he knows that it can't be true because it makes you scream and beg for it to be rammed even harder. Make sure he knows that you love him even though you are verbally ridiculing him because that is part of the game. He has to know that you cherish him and that you are doing this because you wanted to share something extremely intimate and private with him.

Think back to when you first starting dating and how keen he was to make an impression on you and make you happy. He brought you flowers and gifts and opened doors for you. What happened? What's changed? You relaxed into a comfortable relationship and you started taking each other for granted. It works both ways too. Gradually, the light of romance dulls and the passion goes out of the relationship. If you're lucky, you decide to take matters into your hands and move the relationship up a notch so that you can relight the flame within you both again. To do this, go back to the early days of when you first met and remember how it made you feel when he made you feel special, and how good it made him feel too to see the look of love in your eyes, shining back at him. He probably misses those days too so it shouldn't be too difficult to get him to work with you to rekindle that passion. You can bring back those days when you couldn't get enough of each other's bodies, those days when you just wanted to cuddle up in bed and forget the rest of the world. And then life took over.

You probably never gave it a second thought about how much power you held over your partner then and how easy it was to get him to do what you wanted. You still have that power but perhaps he needs reminding of it. And perhaps you do too. You are a very sexual being and you need to be proud of that and make sure everyone else notices of the pride you have in yourself. Visit your hair salon and ask for a style that makes you smile and feel good about yourself when you come out. Buy yourself some new make-up; perhaps have a facial and a massage. Get some new clothes, nothing too tarty but something classy, which enhances your natural body shape and makes the most of what you've got. High shoes are always a turn on for men and make women feel sexy as soon as they slip into them. Even if they do make you wince a little, you don't have to wear them for long or walk a marathon in them; have them on until you get the desired effect, which shouldn't take long.

Be thankful for your sensuality and your sexuality and make the most of it. You are a sexy woman who has the power to dominate men in whichever way she chooses. Make your partner's eyes pop open with anticipation and surprise. Make him remember what he saw in you in the first place. Make his heart race and get him to remember how much he wanted to please you then and how you want him to do the same for you now. You don't have to play the equivalent of the vampy female predator. Just be sure about who you are and what you want. Make men's heads turn. This doesn't mean you have to wear skimpy clothes or flaunt everything you have in the shop window. Sexiness is more about self assuredness and confidence; it's about being happy to be who you are because you like yourself very, very much and know how much you have to offer the world. It's about being the best you that you can be. Tone flabby bodies up, hone dull brains, get off the sofa and do something that interests you. Who would be interested in a drab looking lump of lard who isn't interested in anything but TV? Would you? And when you have shaped yourself into someone you are proud to be, you actually need no one else to tell you how beautiful you are because you already know. And you know how much you can offer your partner if he complies and is willing to help you bring back the excitement into your relationship. If he isn't, then there is something seriously wrong and you need to work on it and start asking questions urgently.

Listen to the answers because whatever he might fob you off with will have a kernel of truth in it and there is usually a way that you can bring things back on track. And when you get there, don't ever forget how close you came to the edge. Make him realize how lucky he is to have you. He may no longer be exactly the man you wanted, nor the man who you first got together with, but if you work at it, he can come very close to it again or even better and you'll end up with a new improved version.

If you're still in the first stages of your relationship, then you should have no doubt about what I'm saying. This early in the relationship you should be heady with love and having wild nights of passion when you are both eager to please each other with your sexual prowess. Can you imagine it ever being any different? Well, it will be unless you always treat your relationship as being precious and nurture it every day. Sometimes that means that you have to lead your partner gently in a direction without him even realizing it's happening. You have a very powerful gift. Use it well and instead of losing it over time, learn how to cultivate it and use it to its best advantage and its fullest capacity.

Relationships inevitably change as time passes. They should grow deeper with each person developing a greater understanding and love for the other person. If you're lucky, this should evolve naturally, but there might be a bit of pushing and shoving along the way until the dominant party rises to the top. This should be done from a stance of loving and caring and it is important to retain that feeling, however explorations fare along the way. Within a loving partnership, it might become irrelevant that you are the dominant party and quite without anyone noticing over the years, it may evolve naturally. It's up to you as a couple how far this invades your lives together. Nothing is written in stone and if you do try something that you feel you will never be able to survive, stick with it. As long as you truly love your partner, there is nothing that your partnership cannot survive and you can always find a way through.

What is Your Role as the Dominant Woman?

If you have developed the right mindset then adopting your role of a dominant woman should not present much of a problem. It's all a matter of confidence and knowing your partner and his desires. However, even though you assume the role of dominant woman does not mean you have to deny that sometimes you might need support to make decisions too. You are a dominant woman, not a superhuman. The role of dominant woman should feel natural after a while but it doesn't necessarily demand that you deny your true self just that you have strong expectations of the way you are treated by others, especially your partner.

Nor does it mean that you should make your partner's life a misery. He wants to continue to respect you and adore you. You don't have to make him terrified to achieve his wish to serve you and make you happy. His primary wish is to *make* you happy and that springs from his love. Of course, there are degrees of sexuality to be discovered almost on a sliding scale. While some men want to be completely dominated in all spheres of their lives, others are more satisfied to be able to serve their partners so that it passes almost without notice by the outside world. While one man might want to be tied down and have to submit to pain which ranges from mild to excruciating, another man might consider this type of treatment way beyond the realms of what might turn him on. Just because you are the dominant person in the partnership does not make you responsible for deciding exactly what will and what will not happen. This should always be a joint decision. He may begin to depend on your authority and look for you to make all important decisions and you might appreciate this but sometimes it is going to be necessary for you to consult with him to help you find a way through difficult problems. Remember that you are his partner, not his mother, although it might sometimes feel to one or both of you that you are. Some men even end up calling their partner's mom by mistake or design, but the very fact that they do speaks volumes.

If you find that your partner actually wants to embrace a full S&D sexual relationship, then you might be so excited that everything happens spontaneously. Alternatively, you may have to give some thought about how to make sure that you both get something worthwhile out of it. Explain that you have not got much experience either and ask him how he wants to approach it. It might be that he wants you to dress up in leather and have the full domme regalia: high boots, leather Basque, stockings. You have to offer him something back that he wants so that he feels happy to participate in what might seem to be an outlandish demand at first. But if you listen carefully and take note of his wishes, then you don't have to be too open about how you will reward him. By him not knowing when, or if, he will be rewarded for his efforts might make it even more exciting an experience, one which he will be more willing to repeat. Do your research. A session might go like this:

He arrives home from work to find you in full domme gear. You are standing with a hand on your hip and your legs are splayed and your head tilting, a cruel and calculating look on your face.

"Where have you been roach?"

(Make time for him to take it all it and be prepared for his mouth to drop open in amazement.)

"I've been at work, you know where I've been. Wh.... What the hell is going on here?"

"Don't ask me questions, you little toad. Come in and shut the door. And for god's sake close your mouth. You look like a real cretin!"

(At this stage there might be total bemusement, even amusement, depending on how much you've discussed previously. At this stage, you are just *feeling* your way and finding out what feels comfortable, so you should both be prepared to feel a little silly at first getting into role.)

"And address me as Mistress, if you know what's good for you. Say it, say it now."

"I've been at work Mistress."

"Hurry up and come in. I want you to remove your

clothes and go to the bathroom."

"Yes, Mistress."

"Call me when you are in the bathroom and completely naked."

When he calls make him wait for a while for you. If he leaves the bathroom, say something like,

"How dare you leave the bathroom without my order? And I heard you the first time. I hate it when you shout. I am not deaf. Now go back to the bathroom and wait there for me naked. And do not let me finding you sitting down. We'll see if there is anything we can do with that sad excuse for a cock."

"Yes, Mistress."

Let him wait for as long as you like and when you can't stand it any longer, go and join him. If he is standing up, go to join him. Take something long, maybe a wooden spoon. If he is standing up and his penis is flaccid, lift it up with the spoon.

"What do you call that sad excuse? It's laughable."

"It's my cock. Mistress."

"Sad. Don't let me see you getting an erection or there will be consequences. Do you understand?

"Yes."

"Yes, what roach?" Tap him lightly on the penis with the spoon.

"Yes, Mistress. Sorry, Mistress."

"Bend over. Hold onto the edge of the bath. I want to inspect you."

Pull his butt cheeks apart and stick your spoon into his anus about an inch.

"Oh you like that do you roach. Well, we had better stop that if you are enjoying it. We're not here for your enjoyment. You must get yourself ready to please your Mistress. Do you agree?"

"Yes, Mistress."

"Get into the shower now roach."

Run the shower on cold and make him stand there under it.

"Well clean yourself roach. Or do I have to hose you down in the garden?"

"No, Mistress."

Pass him some sort of brush, nail or a brush you might use to clean the bath or even toilet.

"Scrub roach. (Pause) Harder. We want all the crap off you if you are coming near me, don't we roach?"

"Yes, Mistress."

"Good, keep it up. You are pleasing your Mistress. Okay, you may get out now. Bend over so that I can inspect you again."

Again, part his cheeks and inspect his anus, sticking the spoon up a bit further and maybe moving it gently around. Smack his ass and tell him to go and stand in the bedroom and wait for you. Make him wait a little while; perhaps you could have a coffee while he's waiting. When you join him, if he is not standing up waiting, punish him by hitting his ass with a spoon. Try and get the bit where the fleshy part meets the back of the leg so that it doesn't leave marks or cause too much pain to start with. Then lie down on the bed and pull your pants/thong to one side and call him over to you.

"Come here roach, and get between my legs. I want you to lick my pussy until I tell you to stop."

Get him to do this until you are satisfied. When you are, tell him to go stand in the corner facing the wall and leave him there for a while. When you are ready, call him over and repeat the same exercise, as above. Have a little snooze if you feel tired.

"That was okay roach. Did you like it too?"

"Yes, Mistress."

"Perhaps I might give you a little treat roach. Would you like that?"

"Yes, Mistress, yes please."

Get into your favorite position for sex.

"Come and make me nice and wet roach. You know what I like."

When you are wet enough and ready for sex, say,

"Okay roach, your time for a little treat. Fuck me now."

Try not to let him come. You can achieve this by squeezing his penis or stopping him intermittently. You can just order him not to come until you say so but this might be for when you are more experienced. If he does climax when you have told him not to however, then you can punish him again.

"Well, that was okay considering the size of your cock. But I think you are going to need much more training. What do you think of that roach?"

"I am very grateful to you Mistress. I am here to serve you."

"Of course you are. Now go run me a bath with some nice bath oil in it."

Have him wash you down and offer up your tits to be massaged with oil and ask him to rub some between your legs. When you are ready, get out of the bath and go and make yourself comfortable on the bed telling him to follow you. Lie on the bed with your legs apart and your knees bent and put your hand between your legs and rub until it feel good.

"Oo, that needs shaving. I want you to shave my pubes roach. Go and fetch the things you're going to need. And do not keep me waiting or you will be severely punished."

When he has finished, instruct him to clear everything away and then come back and lick/fuck you again until you are satisfied. When you are satisfied, tell him it wasn't quite up to your standards so that you think you are going to have to punish him so that he will try harder next time. Tell him to get on all fours and put a dog collar on him with a lead. Lead him to the other side of the bed and secure the lead to something so that he can't just run off. Spank him either with your hand or with another tool, perhaps something that you can use as a paddle this time. Try and find out the optimum level of pain he can withstand but not too hard the first time.

"Stand up. Go into the bathroom. You need another cold shower before you sleep."

"No, please Mistress. Not so cold. And I am hungry and thirsty."

"How dare you! Get in there now. I am going to make you very sorry. Never disobey me again!"

Proceed to give him a cold shower and tell him to remain silent. After a while (don't leave it too long) get him out and paddle his ass for answering back and disobeying. Take hold of the lead and take him to the kitchen.

"Okay, roach. Make me a nice chicken club sandwich and some nice frothy coffee. And it had better be the way I like it. Or else."

After you have finished eating you can allow him something to eat.

"Oh yes, you're hungry and thirsty too aren't you roach?"

"Yes, Mistress."

"Okay, well I'm not all bad. Get Rover's water dish. I will allow you to clean it and fill it with water. Now I think there are some scraps of chicken left so put them in another bowl and put them next to the water on the floor. Okay, down boy. You may eat and drink now."

Give his lead a gentle jerk. When he has finished tell him to clear up and put things away.

"Okay, time to settle down for the night. Go and use the bathroom and then come and see me in the bedroom."

When he joins you in the bedroom, tell him to bend over and inspect his anus again before inserting a butt plug or something that can serve as one. Smack his ass and take him by the lead to a cushion at the side of the bed.

"Down boy. This is where you sleep now until I say otherwise. Down!" Tug on his lead to make him get down on the cushion. Throw a blanket over him and

go about your business.

Obviously this is just a suggested scenario and, of course, you must adapt it as you see fit and so that you feel comfortable with it. Hopefully, you have remembered to discuss with your partner the things that both of you would like to do and you will grow into your role in your own fashion over time. Also, don't forget to refresh your minds with your safe word. If you break down into a fit of giggles at first, don't let it put you off. It should be fun too but hopefully you will learn to uphold your stern and dominant persona over time so that it becomes convincing.

When you have been doing this for a while in your sex life, you might notice that it spreads to other parts of your life, almost without either of you realizing. You might suddenly discover that you are now instructing him on what to do and he is not objecting; in fact, he seems to be relishing his diminished responsibility for taking decisions and handing everything over to you, his Mistress, the woman whom he worships and adores.

What is not to like for you? You get everything done to your standards around the house – this is his punishment and the way he earns your favor. Make the most of it. If you do need to consult him on anything, you can always make it sound as if you are doing him a favor by letting him make a decision for once. Encourage him to show his softer side. You hold all the power. You always have done but you are now learning how to use it to its utmost capacity.

Enjoy!

PART TWO: UNDERSTANDING MALE SEXUALITY

Defining Domination

The image of a leather-clad and booted dominatrix standing over a cowering man is ubiquitous in popular culture. She usually has some kind of torture instrument in hand, a whip, chains, something denoting her status as the S in S&M. With the proliferation of the internet, finding a willing participant in this kink has been made so much easier with many established pro-Domme businesses that offer the service. The question we are going to answer here, however, is what makes a man want to pay for the privilege of being hurt and humiliated or even enter into a relationship with this dynamic in mind? What is the attraction of male submission and what does it mean to be dominated?

Some men report that their fantasies of pain and punishment began when they were very young. It may have started by using pain as a distraction from loneliness or parental neglect. Others developed the kink as a result of juvenile games they played with girls, which involved spanking in role play. Games such as an owner and her misbehaving pet. In this way, the guy discovers that he enjoys it when a girl spanks him. As the boy matures, the nature of the games might differ, but the result remains being spanked by a woman in some way.

Others explore their submissive side by visiting professional dommes and getting to experience being tied to a chair or bed and beaten. At first, the pain, shock, and horror might overshadow the pleasure, but the result is a wave of pain and endorphins that the male submissive finds intoxicating.

This might be a result of masochism rather than submission and this type of male will prefer pain to humiliation. The concept is difficult to explain to someone who hasn't lived it, but it has to do with the intimacy of giving up control to the Domme. It opens the male up to the experience of extreme sensations at the Domme's hands. These extreme sensations provoke clarity of focus in a bid to master them leading the male sub to a floating subspace of accomplishment from having survived the session.

For an inexperienced male wanting to try out submission with a professional Domme, it is recommended that they ask for an introductory session where different aspects of BDSM are introduced to them at the most basic level. This way, they'll be able to discover what they like, and what they don't and where they want to go from there.

A satisfied customer of a Domme reported that he felt the need to please her since she genuinely enjoyed what she did and ensured that he got the experience he desired. Some men do not view being spat on or pissed on as humiliating. Rather it's a personal and intimate act, which they feel honored to have performed on them. It is exactly what they are looking for. Others enjoy having a more sensual domination experience from a Domme who cared about them. Sensual dominance is often depicted as mild or soft using the tools that many vanilla couples use to 'spice things up' such as ropes, feathers, ice cubes, and blindfolds. Role-playing and foot worship are also aspects of sensual dominance.

The male sub will be treated with reverence and praise instead of hurt and humiliation. Even when mild pain is on the menu, it's never the main focus of these scenes but rather a complement to pleasure. Pain is not meant as a means to push the submissive to his limits. It's a great way for couples to experience greater freedom and intimacy. In the opinion of many sensual dominance practitioners, this style of domination needs additional skill sets when it comes to patience and understanding of both what turns the submissive on and his state of mind. This is facilitated by open communication before beginning the scene so as to make sure it is enjoyable for both parties. Even though the pain employed in sensual dominance might be mild, a safe word is still advisable so that the submissive has an out should things get uncomfortable.

Whether it's a professional or a life partner, the important thing to remember is safety first.

Male Submission

The reasons for a male to seek a Domme are as varied as each person. Some men do not claim any psychological trigger for it but put it down to a general desire to please women, especially when their work situation has them in a dominant role all day. The type of submission they seek is also varied. One might want to take part in a cuckold session where they are forced to watch the mistress having sex with another man and then compelled to clean up after them. Such a man would glean pleasure from watching the mistress enjoy herself and relish his role as 'forced' watcher.

In BDSM the male submissive partner also known as a male sub is referred to as the servant. Their Domme in this scenario, which is the dominant partner, is known as femdom. A dominatrix is a woman who is the dominant in BDSM scenarios. Her sexual orientation does not limit the genders of submissives she can partner with. Her role includes but is not limited to the infliction of physical pain. It may simply involve verbal abuse, assigning the submissive tasks that are humiliating or being served by the submissive in any way she chooses. Typically the term dominatrix is associated with a paid professional or pro-domme. The non-professional femdom is usually known as the Domme, coined from a pseudo-French variation of "Domme."

When you make an appointment for role-playing, this

is known as a session and usually takes place in a dedicated play space set up with specialist equipment. This place is labeled as a dungeon. A remote session can also take place by phone or online. Apart from a dominatrix, the dominant partner might also be addressed as Mistress, Lady, Herrin, Goddess or Madame. This creates or maintains the atmosphere in the scene.

Sexual intercourse as well as other intimate acts may or may not feature in the scene with the Domme. This is because Dommes and prostitutes are not interchangeable; their roles differ even though some overlap might exist. Many Dommes are graduates from prestigious universities. Professional Dommes take pride in their ability to read their clients and perform the more technical aspects of BDSM such as extreme bondage, torture role play, Japanese shibari or corporal punishment. These more complex scenes require a greater level of know-how and competency in order to be carried out safely and with the maximum amount of satisfaction to the client.

Financial domination is another scene that some dominatrices play. It's also known as findom and is a fetish where the submissive gets aroused by the act of sending gifts or money to the dominatrix at her command. This can extend to the dominatrix having control over the male sub's finances or they could role play blackmail scenarios. In this kind of scene, the Domme and sub are not in the same physical space. Interaction takes place over the internet.

The types of activities that are considered submissive for men vary geographically and culturally as well as within the context of a specific encounter. For vanilla couples, just having the woman on top during sex might be considered to be submissive to the male. However, in the dominant/submissive relationship, the male sub might manifest in other ways including sadomasochistic sex or servitude that is non-sexual.

Attributes of submission are also used to put the male sub in his place. This involves the symbolism of having on a slave collar made of leather or steel. The dominant might lock him in a chastity belt to symbolize that the male sub has given up all power over his sexuality to the Domme.

Other fun toys used to denote the status of the submissive might include gags, muzzles, and head masks. There is also a SM etiquette to be followed. Some femdoms and their male subs enter into contracts in which the male sub agrees to submit to the femdom. This means they cede themselves to the superior will and guidance of the Domme. This includes being trained, dominated, guided and punished according to the desires of the Domme for a fixed period of time. The male sub agrees to be under the femdom's complete control except under specifically stated limitations. They also agree to adorn their body with the femdom's marks of ownership and wear any restrictive or intrusive objects she might desire up to and including clothing.

They also undertake to prove their virtue to their Mistress such as trust, honesty, obedience, loyalty, and respect. Proof of obedience is required via photos, inspections, and written confirmations. Failure to adhere to these virtues is punished by the Mistress as she deems appropriate.

The male sub undertakes to provide physical, emotional, spiritual and intellectual pleasure after they have undergone training. Limitations to the power of the Mistress might involve the fact that any punishment meted out to the male sub should not cause permanent physical harm and they should also not be detrimental to his career. These rules are not hard and fast and can be modified by mutual agreement.

There is a myriad of ways that male submission can manifest in a relationship. Indeed there are as different ways as there are relationships. However, there are some primers that are common in enforcing male submission. These include:

- Arousal and denial: a great motivator to spur the male to submission is the prospect of denial of orgasm. When the dominant works them up to a state of arousal and then denies them orgasm, they will do absolutely anything she wants.

- Ashtray service is when the male sub acts either as the ashtray or holds the ashtray for the dominant.

- Body worship and service involves rewarding the male sub with the dominant's body. The dominant holds the complete power to bestow or deny the male sub access to her body and thus holds the reins of sexual satisfaction for him.

- Butt plugs can be worn in public and are an excellent medium of control and public humiliation.

- CFNM is an acronym that stands for clothed female, nude male. A naked person is very vulnerable and subject to shame and/or embarrassment in public. Some Dommes use this technique to remind the male sub of their superiority.

- The male chastity belt is a device used to restrict orgasm. Sometimes, no device is used when the male sub is sufficiently disciplined. They are simply ordered not to come and they do it. This does not work for every male sub, however.

- Cock and Ball Torture refers to many actions and devices that cause pain or restrict the genitals in any way.

- Cock rings are also known as the hidden collar. There are so many variations of this device that it is impossible to list them all. Their main function is to control the male sub and mark him as belonging to a certain dominant.

- Corporal punishment is the most common type of BDSM technique in both sexes and involves spanking or caning using various implements from hairbrushes to cat o' nine tails. To add a bit of humiliation to the punishment, the male sub might literally be bent over the dominant's knee to receive his punishment.

- Cuckoldry is a scene where the male sub watches as his Domme gets sexual pleasure from another man while he is forced to watch and denied sexual relief.

- Emasculation happens in various ways when the domme takes away or reduces the male sub's masculinity.

- Female supremacy is a belief system in which females are superior to males.

- Financial control stems from the concept of 1950s housewife where the man would work and then come home and hand over his check to his wife. It's also known as findom as earlier stated.

- Forced feminization is cross-dressing a man who is not a cross-dresser. It is a form of humiliation or embarrassment or could be a kink of the domme. Sometimes it involves something as simple as making him wear panties under his work clothes.

- Goddess worship is similar to female

supremacy, but in this case, the woman is worshipped by her male sub as a goddess or representation of Mother Earth.

- House hubbies can be a permanent thing in the male sub relationship or something that is practiced on the weekend. It involves role reversal where the male subs take on all the designated femme roles in the house.

- Humiliation is a scene that has many forms and types. Some of the most common types of humiliation are physical, verbal and public. Using embarrassment for humiliation is commonly practiced.

- Induced orgasms mean that the domme supervises while the male sub masturbates himself while she gives him instructions and restrictions at will. An example is that she could whip him thirty times while he masturbates and at the thirtieth stroke, he is to come. If he fails to comply the process begins again until he does as he's told. This is a great opportunity for the dominant to get creative and keep things interesting.

- Male milking is another way to control orgasm. The dominant is the one that takes the orgasm from him while he has no control over himself.

- Mounting involves tying up the male sub and then the dominant uses his body as she wishes.

He exists only to give her pleasure.

- Nectar ingestion is the ultimate reward for the male submissive. It involves swallowing the dominant's come.

- Schedule control is when the femdom has complete control over the male sub's time. Telling him what to do and when and giving him specific times that he is to check in.

The Male Sub vs. the Bottom

Many female dominants report that a genuine male sub is hard to find. This is because there is an element of selfishness to some male submissives in that they seek a dominant that can fulfill their fantasies without reciprocity.

While the services of Pro Dommes are eagerly sought and they certainly do see a lot of business, the Dommes usually glean a certain level of dissatisfaction from the interactions because the submissive is interested only in fulfilling their own fantasies without the possibility of compromise in order to take the Domme's desires into account. So while the males define themselves as submissives, they are actually not obedient to the wishes of the dominant and are therefore more accurately referred to as bottoms.

An example of this would be a male sub that wishes to be whipped but does not want to give up the authority to the Domme. By his own definition he is a submissive, but in reality, he is a not. He may submit only partially or not at all to the authority of a Domme during a session. This creates confusion because the very definition of a submissive is subverted.

The psychological mindset of these pseudo subs might help to explain their incompatibility with dominant women. The male submissive might be selfish and the dominant would not be interested in a selfish submissive. The selfish submissive can be identified by how he frames his wishes and needs to the dominant and their subsequent interactions. If he is ready to give the Domme a wish list of scenes but shows no interest or care for the desires of the dominant, then he is a selfish sub. There is a lack of self-awareness displayed when the self-declared male sub messages the Domme to let her know that he will do whatever she says when that is not actually the case.

Many male subs have had years of fantasy about how they would like to express their submission, some of which are very detailed and intricate. Some of these men might not want to do anything other than fulfill these fantasies and any dominant that shows a desire to deviate is immediately dismissed. This may not be termed as pure selfishness because the whole purpose of role-playing a scene is to satisfy desire. However, when they show no care for the needs of the dominant, it comes off as off-putting and unattractive. Dominants also have needs and desires which they wish to satisfy as well as satisfying the submissive.

An illustration of this imbalance is depicted as a submissive contacting a dominant to talk about doing a specific scene and when the dominant brings up her own desires, he ignores that and returns the discussion to the specific scene that he wants. This is a selfish sub. A conversation might go something like this.

"I will let you whip my penis with a cat o' nine tails, ten times."

While the language implies submission, the submissive is actually giving a very specific set of instructions to the dominant. Should the dominant reply with, "What if I paddled your ass instead?" Or wants to add or subtract the number of strokes, then the submissive is not open to that or receptive to any compromise.

This lack of ability to take the other party into account is what is deemed to be selfish and the discussion following it would probably be very unproductive unless there is some major serendipity in which the Domme enjoys *exactly* what the sub is looking for.

Having very specific desires is in itself not selfish at all. It is the unwillingness to consider the needs and desires of the other party that make the male submissive selfish and reduces the level of enjoyment of the experience for both himself and the Domme. If as a submissive the male truly does not care about the desires and needs of the dominant, he should be upfront and honest about it so as to reduce the harm that can be caused to a relationship. The best solution, in this case, is to seek a Pro Domme who will fulfill the male sub's desire for a fee and so they will both garner some satisfaction from the transaction.

It is not at all selfish to make sure that as the male sub your needs and wants are addressed, however failure to consider the needs and wants of your dominant is selfish. As the male sub, you have to listen to what your dominant partner wants even though it is not mandatory to agree to it. Having a mutually beneficial relationship demands that you at least try to meet each other halfway.

Getting to Know Your Male Sub

It is far easier for females to meet male subs than it is for males because there are so many more of them around. The domme is a much rarer animal, and men can struggle to find a partner who will be happy in this role and make it is mutually satisfying, offering enjoyment to both parties. One reason for this is that sexuality is partly developed alongside the society in which we live so obviously, historically, in a male dominated society the man would be the dominant partner. As women's status in western society rises then men have relaxed their blatant masculine traits and allowed the softer, more traditionally feminine sides of their nature to come to the fore. They find that it can be hugely satisfying to submit their power to a woman because it is a way of stepping out of a position of control, which might be necessary, in their profession for instance. Many high-powered men such as politicians and empire moguls relish the opportunity of practicing a submissive sex life because it might be the only time they get to relinquish the constant call on them to be in charge. Not only does this then act as a sexual release but as a stress reliever, thus allowing them to escape from their hectic and demanding lives. Conversely, it might be something that reverts to their childhood or adolescence, as we discussed earlier, and the role of being submissive makes them feel safe as well as sexually aroused.

We are all complex beings and when two people come together in a sexual relationship, it is normally a long and fascinating path we must tread to find out whom that other person truly is.

Have you ever seen a couple out for a meal and neither of them speaks the whole way through the meal? How sad is that? No wonder the divorce rate is so high when so many couples don't even make an attempt at communication, never mind at pleasing each other sexually. To have a good partnership, it is always useful that each person in the relationship actually likes the other. It shouldn't be that hard to find something that you both have in common. A shared sense of humor always helps too. If you don't have anything in common, why are you actually even together? You should try and find something quickly and of course an excellent way of doing this is simply by talking. What's his favorite meal, favorite film, and his best holiday? Questions don't always have to be soul-searching but should give you some information about that person who you genuinely want to know. Don't allow your relationship to deteriorate. Look for new ways to liven it up. You presumably got together because you used to have a good time together. Well, relationships are something that have to be worked at constantly or they shrivel and die.

This encompasses sexuality too. You have had a long time to get to know yourself. But do you really understand what you want from a sexual relationship? Before exploring someone else's sexual makeup you should be self aware, at least up to a point. You might already know that you want to take a dominant role in sex or in the domestic or financial arena, but you are not totally sure how to adopt this lifestyle or introduce it sporadically even. Ideally, what you want to achieve is a mutually beneficial relationship where both parties are comfortable trying out their fantasies – or for some, revisiting them. If you are a true domme and not only adopting those characteristics to satisfy your partner, you will already know what you want to happen. Hopefully you have broached the topic with your partner to tell him about what you want to try.

So that you are both on the same track, communication is the key and that needs to be thorough and deep. Is this something that you are introducing him to or is it something you both have in common from the start of your relationship? Any sexual relationship depends on finding out what the other likes but S&D might be considered outside the realms of the norm for many couples or occur in diluted forms that range from being blindfolded or tied to the bed. It is because there is such a wide spectrum of S&D preferences that it must be fully explored and discussed between the couple. Otherwise, it might result in a total rejection at the initial stages. Your partner might even have tried it before, with another partner, and been deterred from doing it again because of a bad experience.

It is unlikely that you will both want to engage in exactly the same form of S&D but if you do, there would probably be no need to read this book. First, think about your own needs to be a domme. Do you know where and how these feelings developed? Can you remember a time of being in control as a child where it gave you a frisson of sexual enjoyment too? If you do know, then you are lucky. Many of us never give a thought to how we end up feeling as we do, but it can be enlightening and throwing light the onto hidden parts of our mind which trigger sexual desire can be illuminating and help to release us from any misguided guilt which we may feel.

We have not discussed guilt yet, which can have an important bearing on sexual practices. BDSM is outside the range of what is considered as normal for many. This could be for a variety of reasons. For instance, some parents even reprimand their small children for touching their genitals and make the child feel dirty for wanting to explore their own bodies.

Imagine what mental damage this could result in when that child is an adult, and how that mindset could impinge upon them having a happy and guilt-free sex life. Set this against feelings of S&D and it will become apparent how far the journey might have to be to achieve freedom from guilt in order to enjoy.

Thankfully, we all – well, most of us - have boundaries that set a moral complex against genuinely hurting others. I'm talking about rape and murder here and we would never want to partake in any such practice. However, that might not stop us from fantasizing about rape and role playing out such a scenario. And being *naughty* can quite easily be incorporated into the sexual domain by adding an extra dimension and stirring our sensual feelings. But this can only be achieved if we allow ourselves to be free of unfounded feelings of guilt that have infiltrated our psyche in the past. You might have encountered such feelings yourself or still struggle with them now. What you want to achieve though is the power for you and your partner to be free to decide what you want as a couple, as a partnership.

For a woman, the strongest sexual organ is the brain; for a man it is much less complex. Nevertheless, men carry with them the same voices in the head from their childhoods and still can be inhibited in many areas of their sex lives. It is possible to change how someone thinks and to build new neural pathways but this is accomplished over time and must be worked on. Doing so with a partner makes it easier because there is that other person to bounce ideas off and receive feedback on inhibitive thoughts that hold people back and which should be discarded.

Obviously, having good communication lines (dealt with in another part of the book) is a prerequisite of getting to know anyone. What might be more important though, when trying to introduce something into your lives, which could be considered as controversial, is to know how to delve into the recesses of the mind and discover unconscious thoughts that are not helpful. So, instead of just saying, "What do you like?" you are probing deeper to provide the answers to questions like, "*Why* do you like this?" Your partner might not even know himself why he feels the way he does; indeed, you might feel the same, and asking each other these questions can have remarkably meaningful results and build a mutual trust that did not exist previously. It can be an emotional experience because we sometimes hide things from ourselves because they have become too painful to face. However, facing up to our fears and acknowledging that they are hurting us, is cathartic and releases us to develop into someone who is not afraid of life and trying out new experiences. This is not just in the sexual arena but across every area of life. It is empowering.

It can be especially difficult knowing how to start or progress with deeply meaningful interrogative questions and can require great skill to do so. You do not want it to sound like 100 questions and it should flow naturally because there should be a deep desire to know the answers. They are very personal and your partner may never have revealed himself so much to anyone before. To speak in this fashion truly is an indication of submitting to you and putting his trust and faith in your compassion, understanding and love. It can give any relationship a stronger bond but within an S&D pairing, it is especially significant. He does not only trust you with his body, but with his mind too. When the two are combined it is a powerful union which stretches into the union between man and woman of course.

The verbal exchange should be a fascinating experiment when you both exchange deeply hidden facts from your own past. This can be an incredibly warm and emotional experience and one or both of you might even cry. Be ready for that. It's very normal. You could be releasing emotions that have previously been locked away in a box somewhere deep inside of you. Be gentle with each other and make the event memorable and meaningful. Set the scene and tell your partner what you want to do, explaining that you want to deepen your relationship and that submission means that that involves both giving yourself in entirety to the other person. Choose a time when you don't you both are relaxed and have plenty of time. You don't want to have your significant conversation interrupted either, so turn off your phones and don't answer the door to any unexpected guests. This time is sacred. A good place to do it might be in bed so that you can easily hold and comfort each other.

I am going to provide a list of suggested questions to give you an idea of what I mean but this is a suggestion only. Hopefully, once you get started your conversation will find its own pace. If your partner decides that this is the opportunity he has been waiting for and that the time is right, you might only have to ask one or two searching questions. If he gets into his flow, all you have to do is listen. Don't interrupt him but show him that you are listening and indicate that is the case from time to time. You don't have to say anything: nod your head or stroke his head as he's speaking. And don't regale him with your story at this time. He is the subject and it is absolutely important that he feels free and easy to speak. Be aware that any interruption might break the momentum so be sensitive about when and if to ask the next question. Right, let's get started. Remember, this is about getting to know the whole man so that you can enjoy a fuller experience and introduce or develop S&D. We're not expecting yes/no answers; we want the fullest possible explanation of his answers that he can give so encourage him to talk and open up as much as he can. Also, try not to read the questions off rote. They are meant as a guideline only and it really shouldn't feel as if you are using a flip chart to tick off your requirements, which would not seem to be conducive to getting someone to tell you their innermost thoughts and feelings. Be sensitive and alert.

Question 1: What is your earliest sexual memory?

Ask him to give as much detail as possible. You want

to know what it was, where he was, how old he was. Was anyone else there? Ask him if he had an orgasm and if not, when was his first? Once he starts, let him finish.

Question Two: When did you decide you wanted to be dominated by a woman? (Obviously, if you have just suggested this to him, the answer might well be, "When you told me you wanted it. And I'm not sure I do." At least if this is the answer you know the base level you're starting from. And it is all a question of compromise and so it helps you to glean more information about what he does and does not want to do. If he does, however, know when he decided, ask him why he thinks he feels like that.

Question Three: How did you get on with your mother when you were little?

Freud might have been right when he said that all sexual impulses relate back to the mother and it certainly seems possible that it does seem to be the case. You want to elicit from him if she was the one to discipline him and if she ever hurt him physically. How did that make him feel? Does he get on with her now? Does she dominate him now? If so, how does that make him feel?

Question Four: Did he have relationships with any other significant females when he was a child?

How did they treat him? Were they dominant? Did he like to be told what to do? If so, why? Did he still feel as if they cared about him? Does he think that he has carried these feelings about women in general into adulthood? How does that make him feel now?

Question Five: Did you date a lot before we got together?

What sort of girl did you go for when you were younger? Was she demure and shy or confident and self assured? Describe the first time you had sex? Was it good? What is your perfect woman – and you don't have to say it is me? Have you ever had a girlfriend who bossed you about and liked to take charge? If yes, how did it make you feel?

Question Six: What is your idea of a perfect sex session?

Do you think you have had a perfect sex session yet or has it still to happen? Describe it in detail? Does it involve oral sex? Who is giving it and who is receiving it? Who is in charge: you or her?

Question Seven: How many women have you slept with before we got together?

Why so many/few? Before me, what was your best sexual relationship? Why? What did you like doing best sexually within that relationship? Was she domineering at all? How?

Question Eight: Do you think you have any fetishes?

What are they? How do you think they developed?

When did you first become aware of wanting to do that?

Question Nine: What do you know about female domination and male submission?

Have you read any books or magazines about it? Have you ever looked it up online? Was there anything that excited you? Describe it in detail? If you think about it now, what sort of thing would excite you? Describe it to me.

Question Ten: What was it that attracted you to me?

Do you think I am the dominant one in the partnership? Would you like me to be more dominant? How would you feel if I was the dominant sexual partner? What would you like me to do to you exactly? Why do you think that that would excite you? Do you like the idea of being submissive and letting me take charge? What areas would you be willing for me to be dominant in? Sexual? Domestic? Financial? All areas? All the time or just part of it? How much? Be very explicit.

Question Eleven: Does the idea of pain during sex excite you?

Explain how you would like to be hurt. Would you like me to spank or whip you? What article would I be using to do so? Do you want to feel vulnerable? How would you feel if you showed me an emotion that indicated a weakness in you or revealed a feminine side in you?

Does it ever feel tiring to be the one in charge all the time? Do you think pain could be pleasurable? What sex aids would you like to use or wear?

Question Twelve: Do you think that women are superior to men?

What makes them better or worse? Do you think that men and women are equal in all respects? If not, how do they differ? Do you think difference is important in a relationship or should everything be decided and done equally? Should men and women have distinct roles? Should this distinction or sameness be carried over into their sex lives? How should it be determined who does what? Should one person get to decide on important things? Should one person get to decide on what happens sexually between a couple? What should happen if I ask you to do something that you don't want to do? How far would you go before you said no? Would you be willing to at least try something new? If not, why not?

Question Thirteen: How do you feel about being verbally abused by me?

Would you like me to mock you physically and demean you? Would you like to feel emasculated? If you think you would enjoy this, why do you think you would?

Question Fourteen: And now, onto physical actions. What do you feel about the following? Do you think that you would like to try them with me?

(This is an opportunity to suggest things that you might want to do and might include the following.) Cock and ball torture; me using a strap-on dildo on you; acting the cuckold and watching me with another man – or woman; being denied an orgasm and just pleasing me until I say you can come too; would you like me to urinate on you: would you like to be publicly dominated; would you wear a butt plug all day; would you let me dominate you in front of other women or men; would you like to be my sex slave; would you like to go to sex clubs and dress up and perform publicly; would you like to be totally submissive to me, either for an agreed time and indefinitely? If he answers yes or no, ask him to explain what turns him on or off about the suggestion.

Question Fifteen: Do you have complete trust in me to do the things that you desire?

Is there anything that I have not mentioned that you think you would enjoy? Tell me about it in detail.

Question Sixteen: Tell me a secret that you have never told anyone else.

Explain that this might be because he has felt ashamed of it ever since it happened. It might be something from his childhood, adolescence or something that happened recently. You have to promise not to be angry or upset. He is asking you to understand anything that he chooses to share with you and trusting you not to treat that information lightly or disrespectfully. How will you feel if he discloses he has had an incestuous relationship for instance? Or that he has cheated on you? There really can be no half measures if he is putting his whole trust in you not to reject him. Before you ask the question, be sure you can cope with the answer.

Of course, these are just suggestions of questions but I hope that they give you the flavor of what sort of thing you should be asking. After you get started on the first one or two you might discover that your partner has been waiting for a long time for you to take control of him and he might gush all his pent-up feelings in one swoop like an unstoppable force, relieved that he is allowed to be himself without judgment from you. It is highly unlikely that you will get exactly the answers that you thought you would but what you should get is a strong indication of how he feels on the topic of female domination. Everything is then up for discussion and there might have to be compromises along the way so that you both get what you want. However, if the partnership is trusting and loving, where both partners want to please the other.

You might decide between you that you would like a bit of both sides and that you want to be free to flip from time to time. You might have a desire to be submissive too and in the initial stages your partner might feel as if he is not ready to totally relinquish the reins to you. It might be a long, slow path until you can try out exactly what you want without him feeling uncomfortable and that it holds no pleasure for him, so have your patience ready in heaps. Of course, by discussing the subject at length you have already got him to open up to you and disclose his most private thoughts. He has already illustrated that he has complete trust in you and now you must show him that his trust is not misplaced. If, during the course of your discussion, has agreed that he trusts you to do certain things to him, start now. If you are on the bed, undress him until he is completely naked. If he is not erect already, then either suck his penis until it is or use your hands to masturbate him. He should be lying on his back and you could perhaps ask him to lick your pussy at the same time. As soon as he is erect, turn around and climb on top of him. You should be fully clothed. Nakedness usually makes us feel more vulnerable and this is the emotion you should evoke. Try and control his climax by slowing down when you sense he is coming and squeeze his balls tightly with your hand. If he winces or cries out, punish him in a way that you have just agreed he is willing to submit to. His orgasm(s) should be orchestrated by you.

Do not do anything, at this stage certainly, which he has not just agreed to. If you cross over that line, then you are instantly negating the whole point of the exercise by instantly betraying his trust. If he seems to be enjoying the experience, elongate it by introducing something else which demonstrates your dominance over him. You might tie him up for instance and maybe blindfold him. You will soon know if this is something that excites him because of the continuity or absence of his erection. Be mindful of what you are doing and try and concentrate on the things that he has said he would enjoy. No doubt you will remember whatever he has said that resonates with your wishes too.

And just because you are adopting the dominant role does not mean you cannot still be a generous lover. A good sexual liaison should be one that pleases both partners and if he is willing to become submissive for some of the time only, and wants to be dominant at others, you should be willing to agree to this also. It is about mutual trust and by answering your questions fully and honestly, he has already demonstrated his trust in you so perhaps you could reciprocate by answering his questions for you. He might want to compose them himself; indeed, he might well have a set of extremely intimate things he wants to try with you that you have not yet touched upon. Try and be as honest as you possibly can.

However, if he really is dismissive then he may be a little shy about asking for what he wants so you could start him off with a list of questions to use as a warm-up. Hopefully, once you start talking intimately, he will gather confidence and start asking his own questions. The important thing to take away from this exercise is that you are encouraging openness between you both and a sense of total trust and empathy. You should both want to please the other, whether you are in dominant or submissive mode. This might be in the same session or be agreed on beforehand. Spontaneity might be preferred or just the fact that you know what and when it is going to happen might add to your titillation.

Just as suggestions, I have added some questions that he might wish to pose to you. If he is feeling nervous about how to get started, then it gives him an advantage of being able to use the questions as a crib sheet. Hopefully, you should both feel comfortable about answering intimate questions after having him answered yours. Try to get him to ask your questions in a different session because it might lead in another direction which is more about his fulfillment rather than concentrating on yours. However, it may still be about pleasing you but it might involve him taking the lead and being the dominant. The questions will of course depend on his preferences and so the ones suggested here might not be at all appropriate but at least he can adapt them for his own requirements.

Question One: How old were you when you lost your virginity?

Did you enjoy it? Who was it with? Was it a one-off or in a stable relationship? Why didn't you wait until you were older? Why did you do it so young?

Question Two: How do you feel about being dominated?

Why do you feel like this? Do you prefer to be dominant? Why (not)?

Question Three: Do you have any fetishes?

Describe them and tell me if you know how they developed?

Question Four: Who disciplined you when you were a child?

Did you have any sexual feelings that surrounded discipline? Did you have sexual feelings towards any male members of your family when you were growing up? If so, what were they?

Question Five: What is your most frequent fantasy?

Would you like to roleplay this? Do any of your fantasies involve more than one partner or lesbian sex? Tell me about them?

Question Six: What is your earliest sexual memory?

Describe it in full detail? Other than full intercourse, what was your first sexual experience? Did someone else instigate it or did you?

Question Seven: Have you ever had an orgasm?

When was it? Describe it to me? Have you ever had multiple orgasms? What makes you come the quickest? What is your favorite sexual position? Do you like anal sex? Do you like to be spanked? Do you like to be blindfolded? Do you like to be tied up?

Question Eight: Do you think that women are superior to men?

If so, how? Why do you think you feel this way? Was your mother a dominant woman? Was your father submissive? Did he treat you like a princess?

Question Nine: Why were you attracted to me?

What was it exactly that you liked about me? Do you like it when I tell you what to do, generally and sexually?

Question Ten: Are you prepared to submit to me completely?

Do you trust me to dominate you completely? How do you feel about female submission? And male submission? Why does male submission appeal to you?

By this stage, you should both feel totally relaxed and comfortable discussing intimate issues. If there has been awkwardness or a relationship imbalance where one person has all the fun and the other has none, this exercise should help to redress the balance. And you are ready to go. So, where do you start? A good place might be to become fully conversant with your partner's body. He might not have been lucky enough to have had a partner who has been willing to please him before so if this is a new experience for you both, so much the better. Pain is usually tempered with exquisite pleasure and the following might give you a few good ideas of what to try out.

Erogenous Zones

The whole point of kink is to give and receive physical, mental and emotional satisfaction and in order to do that, it is pertinent to know how the body works to evoke pleasure and pain. On the male, there are many spots that when stimulated will evoke a pleasurable response. One such spot is the frenulum, which is located at the junction between the glans and the shaft on the underside of the penis directly below the head. The frenulum is described as the male clitoris. It reacts very well to hands and tongue stroking slowly to build arousal.

The soles of a male's feet are more innervated than those of a female. About a third of the way down from the third toe is an acupressure point located right in front of the arch in the foot's center. It's known as the 'bubbling spring' and pressure on it will stimulate circulation throughout the body, arousing him. A foot massage on this point is all you need to get the male going.

The p spot is perhaps the best known erogenous zone on a man. This is the prostate gland, which is found in the anus, about three-quarters of a finger length in and feels like a walnut. It is extremely sensitive due to extensive innervation. A simple massage of this spot is enough to induce orgasm. It can not only be stimulated from inside of the anus but also on the outside at the perineum which is the smooth strip of skin between his anus and balls.

A surprisingly erogenous zone that may be overlooked is the thumb. Sucking on his thumb in a sexy way provokes thoughts of having his penis sucked and this engages his mind and emotions and leads to arousal.

The gluteal fold may be the reason the male sub enjoys spanking so much. This crease between the top of his thigh and his ass is a very sensitive area and guaranteed to provoke arousal.

There is also a triangular bone at the base of the spine known as a sacrum that is also a bundle of nerves said to connect to the genitalia. Stimulation especially of an electrical nature has been known to lead to orgasm.

Nipples are another well known erogenous zone with endless potential for both pain and pleasure. In addition to licking, sucking and biting, nipples can be twisted and pulled or clamped with nipple clamps. The clamps keep blood flow in the area making the nipples even more sensitive and stiff. Ice can be employed to provide a nice contrast in temperature, which heightens sensation.

The scrotal raphe is the line that runs through the middle of the scrotal sack. The scrotal sack covers the balls. Stimulation by licking and application of pressure is arousing and can lead to powerful orgasms.

Prostate massages begin with stimulation where a finger or sex toy is inserted into the anus and gently massage by application of pressure on the rectal wall. If you're doing it right, you'll feel involuntary contractions in the PC muscles and sphincter. There will be a slight sensation of fullness and warmth in the rectum. The area around the prostate begins to increase in tension and warmth. This is followed by trembling, which leads to orgasm, sometimes multiple orgasms as there is no refractory period for prostate orgasms. Lubrication is essential to grease this process along. Without it, this process can be dangerous and painful.

Other ways to stimulate arousal include hand jobs and blow jobs. The former is probably the easiest to do since it simply involves placing a hand gently on his crotch, massaging and rubbing to get him going and getting ever more aggressive with time, grabbing and squeezing his penis before releasing. Using lubrication makes this process run smoother.

Giving a blow job mostly involves using your mouth rather than your hands to stimulate arousal and then possibly letting him fuck your mouth. The frenulum being a really sensitive area is a good place to start with delicate nips and kisses. Gentle teasing is great for prolonging arousal especially as part of arousal/denial play. Licking and sucking follow and then taking his entire dick in your mouth and letting him fuck your mouth. You can flick your tongue up and down and from side to side to stimulate his nerve endings and then rotate in circles to really get him going.

PART THREE: COMMUNICATION AND SATISFYING EACH OTHER'S NEEDS

Open and Honest Communication

Communication is a key ingredient in order to engage in a successful bondage, discipline, sadism, and masochism, relationship. Consent is a primary pillar of the kink and one can't consent to something that has not been discussed. When that kink involves hurting someone in a way that they will enjoy, it is even more pertinent not just to communicate with words, but actions as well. When the Domme is carrying out a whipping or assessing the effects of making the male sub wear a butt plug all day, it is not just his words she must pay attention to, but his body language as well. Being a Domme requires constant alertness to small changes in the male sub's demeanor in order to assess their levels of enjoyment, what's working and what's not. However, this cannot be left to the Domme alone. The sub must speak up if he is unhappy or feels dissatisfied with how a scene is going. Adjustments can be made so that everyone comes away feeling empowered. When a male sub is uncomfortable or unhappy with a scene and just goes along with it in order not to make waves, the results can vary from unsatisfactory to disastrous.

Full transparency is not just a term bandied about on BDSM online forums. It is a necessary ingredient to any relationship especially when there is an owner/property dynamic involved. It is the key to making a relationship work and it is best to begin as you mean to go on.

The male sub is better at articulating his wants and needs than the female submissive, but they could still withhold information because they think that is not what the domme wants to hear. The best way to deal with this fear of total honesty is not to heap blame, but to explain clearly your point of view of what you need from the relationship. This might take more than one attempt to get right, but it is worth it in terms of quality of the relationship. The key is to desire each other's happiness and the health of the relationship through good communication.

The ability to communicate well ties in with the point of view of the male sub and his domme. To begin to answer this question, it is imperative to know whether there is a real difference between male and female submission. Is the former more about mental domination than physical? This question arises because of the mindset that men are stronger than women and therefore women would have to resort to other means to subjugate the male.

This is not necessarily true.

Any attempt to generalize a situation usually results in misunderstandings because they rarely hold water.

Not much is written about the relationship between the femdom and her male sub. So it is difficult to gather data to prove or disprove anything except for the vague conception that this relationship mainly relies on mental dominance.

Physical dominance involves using bondage toys and other means to subdue a sub. This could involve tying them up, whips, chains, physical punishments and impact play, all of which are widely practiced by Dommes and thoroughly enjoyed by male subs. Mental dominance, therefore, would involve everything else such as coming up with a slave contract, having rules and regulations, schedule control, arousal denial, humiliation, objectification, orgasm control, mental bondage and mental chastity along with many other games. In all of these, the domme need not engage in any physicality. For the new male sub or even domme, it is a question worth clarifying in order for expectations to be aligned.

The whole question might arise because of obsolete societal norms where the male is supposed to be the stronger one, the aggressor and so the 'fairer sex' has to resolve to 'female wiles' to get their way. This is a false narrative that has been debunked severally, but questions might still linger. Communication is the backbone of any relationship especially the BDSM one. The way that you choose to communicate can be dictated by whatever guidelines and rules you have in place. The dominant listens to the submissive's needs and strives to fulfill them. In return the submissive cedes all responsibility for their pleasure to the dominant, trusting them to do their best to execute them. Trust goes hand in hand with open communication; you can't have one without the other.

Any d/s relationship begins with mental dominance before progressing to physical dominance. Before the games begin, there must be a desire to submit and a willingness to cede all control to another person and adhere to their rules and regulations including punishments and other consequences. Before someone gets tied up or beat down or worships at the other's feet, mental submission has to have occurred.

BDSM has some things that are truly inherent to this kink and that is the power given to the dominant by the submissive with their consent. The other thing is that domme/subs are some of the best communicators in existence and believe most ardently in feminism and a relationship that is consent-driven. This is because there needs to be maximum respect for each other's views as well as good communication in order to negotiate a BDSM scene. What this entails is setting boundaries and limits, being honest with each other about the each other's levels of comfort and learning to speak up if things go too far.

Dominants may have individual preferences when it comes to mental vs. physical dominance, but this preference is not divided by gender. Most d/s relationships tend to cover the entire spectrum of dominance and the best femdoms do so with mastery and skill. Being able to flog a sub is one thing, but to do so while fucking with their mind at the same time is even better. There is no proven area that belongs to one gender more than another. There is very little in the BDSM lifestyle that belongs exclusively to one gender, but if you are uncomfortable with any aspect of the kink, open communication is the key to a happy life.

The only aspect of play that really has some gender bias is cuckolding simply because by definition it involves a man's partner having sexual relations with someone else while their mate watches and he is denied. Sissification or feminization is another aspect that could have this gender bias simply because there is no such thing as masculinization of female subs.

The reasons why men would be interested in the submissive lifestyle vary according to reports. In some cases, it has been found that most men in positions of social power are more likely to be submissive in bed. This is because those positions reduce inhibition. Inhibition is a feeling that makes one self-conscious and unable to act in a relaxed and natural way.

Thus, when he finally gets the opportunity to have sex, he would prefer the role of "submissive."

According to reports males also exercise submission in order to express their masculinity. Some men went as far as to say that they had never felt manlier than when they felt pain hence they are willing and happy to take part in submissive practices in bed. They feel that the more pain they can endure the more manly or masculine they are. Many men are feminist and believe in the empowering of women and most if not all women are feminist and they believed in the reversal of roles in the household. They believe that women shouldn't just have to stay home and take care of the family. The same is in bed they believe that women could and should dictate in between the sheets as well. They have a need to be the dictator just to prove to society that she can wield power and the man agreeing with her is very submissive and follows orders as issued to him. Reports have shown that such relationships come to be as weak men, not necessarily physically but also mentally, have a need to be with women who are strong, independent and with an urge to hold power. These women complete these men. Other men whom may end up being submissive are 'momma's boys.' Reports show that these men are used to having a strong female presence running their lives hence they seek women whom would run their lives even up to the local level of the bed.

Being a submissive is associated with some hard to deny qualities such as being eager to please and looking for validation in the dominant. The submissive is compelled to place their power and trust in someone else's hands. It is not a trait that can be wished away or fades with time, although the submissive can choose to nurture it. This is different from training someone to become a submissive.

Many people view the BDSM relationship as a difficult one to maintain. However, this may not necessarily be true because of the pre-negotiated rules and boundaries that exist between the domme and the sub. The submissive expects that he can surrender himself to the dominant and trust her to do everything to look after him.

All he needs to do is obey.

Many submissives find this to be a very relaxing aspect of their relationship. They know what the domme expects from them and where they belong and knowing what is expected removes the guesswork and thinking out of everyday activities. The act of submission is not limited to sex roles. It consists of everyday things that the sub does for the domme if they are in a relationship, which makes the sub feel important. This includes things like being the house hubby, goddess worship or wearing slave collars or cock rings.

Submissives are subject to schedule control, must remain obedient, and take on punishments for transgressions against their accepted rules and boundaries should the domme choose to compel them to. Punishment might entail cleaning tasks specifically set up or wearing a plug for a long time – this is because, in the short term, a plug is pleasurable as it hits against the prostate. This is because of the plethora of nerve endings present in that region. However, for long periods of time, it might start to get uncomfortable.

It is not just rules and regulations that govern the domme/sub relationship. This type of relationship only thrives if both partners feel that there is trust, honesty, and communication flowing between them. Especially for the submissive that submits themselves to the mercy of the dominant, they need to feel that they can trust them implicitly. Without that, the relationship cannot be sustained. Even when the male sub visits a Pro Domme, there is still the necessity of trust in the relationship in order for them both to enjoy the scene. This is why she advertises her services in a very specific manner and has extensive discussions with clients beforehand on what they need from her and vice versa.

The domme/sub relationship involves things like being tied up and gagged. Without trust, on both sides, honesty, respect, and communication, this can lead to some dangerous situations.

It takes a lot of courage to be totally honest with each other, but the rewards are worth stepping out of your comfort zone in order to fully comprehend each other's wants and needs completely. Communication is the key to honesty. When you are able to articulate your needs clearly and have the other person listen and understand that is the beginning of trust. The BDSM relationship does not mean that the submissive's wants and needs are not as important as the Domme's. The sub can say no and discuss their needs with the domme in order to make the experience enjoyable for both of them.

To be a sexual submissive is not the same as being a submissive in every aspect of life. In fact, some submissives are quite loud and aggressive in their places of work and in everyday life. But when it comes to the sexual relationship, they're docile and want to be told what to do.

For some, BDSM is about kink. They subscribe to all of the various kinks that are characteristic of the lifestyle. Others only subscribe to some of the kinks of the BDSM lifestyle. The domme/sub relationship is usually distinguished from sadomasochism by the difference in power dynamics between the couple. The domme/sub relationship is characterized by the domination of one over the other. A person who identifies as being in a domme/sub relationship probably has an aspect of power play present in their sexual life.

Boundaries

There are certain issues that must be considered when adopting a BDSM lifestyle and it is important that safety measures are implemented to ensure optimum enjoyment. Mostly, it is common sense, but the topics below deserve mention. It goes without saying that pain should have agreed upon levels and that no one should suffer more pain than he or she is willing to submit to. It can sometimes be a fine line and that is why it is so important that explicit guidelines are discussed and agreed upon beforehand. You will have to experiment to establish what pain threshold can be sustained, and how much energy you have to keep you going.

Some issues will be personal to you of course. Perhaps one of you is physically disabled and must make adaptations for you both to enjoy the practice of S&D but there is no reason why the pleasure should be completely denied and most problems can be overcome with a little thought and effort.

Also, bear in mind that we all feel differently at different times so that you should discuss before each session what you find acceptable at any particular point in time. It might be that something you did last time is not what you want at all this time. Ask your partner to be clear about this from the start and make your own wishes known too. Assumptions can be a dangerous thing. It is advisable to agree on variations on a theme so that what you do does not become too predictable or you could be slipping into the same sort of habits just with different actions. Be ready to change things around a bit and take ideas where you can find them.

Protecting the Children

It almost goes without saying that your S&D behavior should not be overt or that children should be exposed to any facet of it, and that includes equipment. There is already legislation in place to protect children and exposing a child to something that they are not emotionally equipped to deal with would come under this heading. Try and be mindful of what you are saying in front of children and of your actions. If you do use sex toys or equipment, keep them tightly locked away and out of view. Remember, that a child's curiosity will only be piqued by a locked box, and if the key is available, who could really blame them for investigating? A flimsy lock would not be a good idea either. And don't even think of having a sex room or dungeon in your cellar! The best way is to keep your S&D sessions for when the kids are away on a sleepover or when you can persuade grandparents to look after them for the night. They might take them home for the night or you could book into a cozy and remote cottage, somewhere that allows you both to make as much noise as you wish without disturbing anyone or making the neighbors' curtains twitch.

Privacy

Talking about privacy, although your sexual practices are no-one's business but your own, some people would love to be privy to your juicy sex life to brighten up their own dull existences. If you live in a small town, it might be especially difficult to keep your private life private so be careful who you confide in. Be careful not to have any boozy nights where you decide to open up to someone and tell all. The chances are that you will deeply regret doing so the next day. Make a pact with your partner who and who will not be allowed to know about your private life.

If you live in a big metropolitan area, do not assume that this makes you anonymous either. It is amazing how easy it is to go to the other side of the world on vacation and still run into two people you went to school with. So unless you want your sex life to be public knowledge keep your mouth tightly shut. Imagine how your children would feel if they heard at school that their mom said you were perverts.

Also, be very careful if you are considering appearing in sex magazines where the readers send in their own or their partner's photos as donations to be included in the publication. The same thing applies to putting photos online too. Yes, it can be extremely horny to imagine thousands of other people looking at you or your partner and salivating over the sight of him. But unless you want to be regarded as a freak by the locals – or worse still your mother whose neighbor brought it to show her for her own good – then keep away, and keep your bodies for each other's eyes and delectation only.

Safe Word

If you intend to partake in S&D, one of the first things that you should decide is a safe word. Make this something out of the ordinary; do not choose something you might use in everyday conversation and certainly not *STOP,* however vehemently. Make it something like banjo or someone's name, but something that you both recognize as a true red light stop sign. You must never ignore this word and you must both agree that it is to be used only when you truly mean it. Otherwise, it loses its effectiveness and is no longer safe.

Health and Safety

This is of paramount importance and must always be regarded as number one priority. It can be fatal if you ignore basic rules about safety in the heights of passion. If, for instance, your partner has something around his neck to secure him, and you are pulling the other end, he may not be capable of even shouting out the safe word if you are slowly choking the life out of him. The objective of this type of role play can be so that the submissive feels that his partner is in total control and there is some association with being attached to a lead and treated like an animal perhaps, which is a form of degradation. However, sometimes this is used as a way to restrict breathing and if it is restricted too much then the sub could pass out or even be killed unintentionally. Please be extra careful when using this form of domination.

It can also almost go without saying that erotic asphyxiation is probably one of the most dangerous practices in the realm of BDSM. This is where the brain is deprived of oxygen to add to sexual sensations. This might be achieved by putting a plastic bag over the head. Deprivation of oxygen and the build-up of carbon dioxide within the bag can result in a feeling of giddiness, pleasure and light-headiness. When this feeling is combined with orgasm people report that it is better than snorting cocaine and it is hugely addictive. This was first discovered in the 17th century during hangings. Spectators noted that when men were hanged they very frequently developed erections which even remained after the man was dead. Some were even known to ejaculate. There are many incidences of accidental death and it would not be advised to try this at all, even if you consider yourself to be a medical expert. If killing someone gives you pleasure, then this is definitely not the book for you. In fact, the book for you has probably not been written yet.

If one or both of you are suffering from health problems then you must adapt what you do. Vigorous sex has been known to kill a fair number of people. But what a way to go! If it is the male partner who is not very mobile or suffers from heart problems maybe, it may even be advantageous for the woman to take the dominant role and be on top during intercourse. He can still please you with oral sex or sex toys such as vibrators too. It's just finding a way to be inventive around what pleases you both and is not detrimental to anyone's health.

Always remember to be hygienic. Some people have expressed that they like their partners to like out their ass holes after going to the toilet, or drink their urine. The first one is not advised because they are imbibing thousands of bacterial particles which could make them very sick and even cause hepatitis or liver failure. Drinking urine is a little more acceptable and people have been known to avoid dying of thirst by drinking their own urine. Nevertheless, it is not advisable to drink large amounts or to do it regularly.

Felching may be a lesser known form of this and involves sucking out the semen from the anus. Sucking semen out of a vagina is known as cream pie eating and is probably much less risky. The golden showers should also be reserved for other parts of the body rather than the mouth. While it will probably not prove fatal, it cannot be sensible to gamble with your own or someone else's health. If in doubt, do not do it. Do not imbibe anything that there can be the least bit of doubt about and if you don't have any knowledge about it, research it.

Never put yourself or your partner in physical danger from which he cannot escape. Just like the safe word, he should always have ways to release himself from a potentially dangerous position, if you leave him alone for instance and a fire started because of an electrical fault. Make it possible for him to unlock any locks by leaving a key for emergency use. If he uses it in a non-emergency situation, he can always be punished later for the crime, much more preferable for being prosecuted for manslaughter or unlawful killing.

Another aspect of health and safety encompasses mental health. Experimenting with something new that deeply involves emotions can prove to be extremely unsettling, especially when one person in the relationship does not feel entirely secure to start with. This, in turn, can prove to be detrimental to one's mental health if you are trying to comply with your partner's wishes to please them but it is against your own will and makes you ill. Mental torture should not be ignored but attended immediately to in order to rectify it.

Impact play is about using a palm on another object to spank or hit. There can be toys or objects that your partner does not wish to use and this should be respected. Also, when inflicting pain, be mindful of where on the body you hit them. Hit them on the fleshy part of the bottom and try and avoid any major organs that could easily be damaged. Under no circumstances should you be hitting the stomach or the chest. You should also avoid the sides of the spine which is where the kidneys are sited.

Who's involved?

Agree if you both want to involve other people. Does your partner wish to be a cuckold and watch you having sex with someone else? Only he knows the answer to this question and if this is something that turns you on but he says that it would hurt him considerably, then it may have to be something you agree to forego. A sexual impulse is not worth risking a long-term loving relationship and by agreeing to boundaries you are promising not to step outside of them. Ask him to tell you his reasons and you share yours. However, if a compromise can be reached on this, move onto something on which you both can agree.

Using Drugs or Other Stimulants

When you are participating in BDSM, it is advisable to use drugs, especially hard drugs to enhance the experience. A glass or two of wine might relax you so much that it alters your senses might be unwise and even dangerous. As you know, your perceptions are altered by drugs and alcohol and you lose the sense of how heavily you might be applying pressure or for how long you administer corporal punishment. So lay off over imbibing at least until the session is over and when you can relax and discuss what happened. Don't be tempted into drinking more than you know you can handle or taking drugs that you don't want to because your inhibitions are lowered and when performing S&D you are releasing any control to the person who might be more sober than you. Indeed, what is the point of being so drunk or drugged up that you don't even remember how fantastic your session has just been? Keep it for another time. Maybe for a celebration that your partner has finally come over to the other side and can't wait to be the submissive to your dominant for life.

Pain Thresholds

We all have different capacities for pain. Some women say that they have never felt any pain more intense than childbirth while others seem to have babies like shelling peas. We all feel pain differently and when it is used for sexual purposes, then it should be mixed with pleasurable feelings so that it elicits an exquisite sensation of ecstasy. You may have to experiment with the levels of pain that he can withstand and be drawing upon the safe word incessantly. Alternatively, he may surprise you by being able to withstand immense pain.

Don't belittle him for being cowardly or it might just put him off the idea totally. You have to be very experienced before you can mix physical pain with verbal abuse so go slowly to start with and build up gradually. A submissive should never lie about his pain threshold because he thinks he is pleasing his partner. This is a very risky tactic. Everyone should be encouraged to be honest and say if something is hurting more than they can bear. There is no shame when enjoyment is being marred because the punishment is not being doled out at the required level. There is also nothing wrong in your partner asking for a break so that he – and you - can recoup the energy expounded. Giving and receiving corporal punishment can be hard work. As you become more experienced, you will know your partner's limits. If you think that your partner has had enough, even if he denies that is the case, use your own judgment and stop. You can incorporate this into the role play and make him think that you are leaving him to languish until you are quite ready to resume. Make it seem as if the break or even the cessation is your intention.

Public humiliation

You must agree where the arena for S&D is and how far it stretches. Is your partner comfortable with being publicly humiliated as part of the role play or does he wish to keep it just between the two of you and only acknowledge it when you are in your own home alone. You may decide that you want to visit clubs that specialize in BDSM and this will involve making it public. If he is comfortable with overt public domination, then you can have fun deciding how to dress up. These places are normally way OTT and packed to the rafters with colorful and exotic people. They usually have playrooms which can be set up like dungeons with lots of equipment that is free for anyone to use. People can go here to meet others or just to be exhibitionist with their own partners. The club will offer many opportunities for diversification and variety and it's up to you to choose what you want to be part of. It's always a good idea to be clear about your limitations before you arrive there so that you don't cause a public scene unintentionally. Look the club up online before you commit to going or try and get information on what to expect from someone who has already been. Your visit might be a one-off or you might become addicted and regard it as an extension of your social life. At the very least, you might come away with some interesting ideas to try out at home. But you must both be very clear that it is something that you both want to do.

Using Literature and Porn

It might help you both to decide upon boundaries if you look at porn films on the subject together. These could range from soft porn like Fifty Shades of Grey and then perhaps graduate to something harder. It might be a case of scream when you *don't* want to go faster. Test the water to find out what turns you both on and agree to try it yourselves. You could also try reading some literature on the subject. Buy your partners magazines or books to read on the topic and then ask him when he has finished reading them to tell you about anything he would like to try out. Again, this could generate some interesting ideas.

Definitely Out of Bounds

Discuss in details those things that either of you feel a definite aversion towards. This can be changed at the start of a new session when you are saying what you definitely don't want it. If you overstep this mark, then it could be classed as abuse. You could make this more formal by putting it in writing. As you discuss what you want to do at length with each other, write down columns of yes and no. Both of you must agree to anything you put in the yes column and only one person must be against anything in the no column. You can then sign and date this and if something should happen which your partner disputes and says that he hasn't agreed to this, then you can always refer to the signed contract. This can be changed at any time because there has to be flexibility anyway. One causes ecstasy one day, may cause huge disgust and abhorrence the next so keep this updated and refer to it regularly. New ideas can be added as you go along and they don't have to be totally explicit because it is always nice to have some room for maneuver and an element of surprise. Things would not be half so exciting if your partner knew exactly what to expect. This is more about general boundaries around pain and things that you both find acceptable.

Level of Limits

In the BDSM community, there is terminology that coins the different levels of boundaries set. Hard limit draws a line that must definitely not be crossed. This might be because of a physical injury or disability. A soft limit is something that the sub might agree to but might still feel apprehensive about committing to completely. It is therefore essential that any practices under this heading are approached with caution. A requirement limit is a negotiation, so it might involve a conversation very much like, "If I agree to this, I will need that afterwards." This can all be added to the contract as outlined above.

Finally, remember that there should be no hard feelings afterward about what is agreed or decided upon. If you feel that you very much want to participate in a particular activity and your partner has very strong feelings against it, then please do respect their wishes. Never force someone to do anything. It can be very easily sold to a willing partner as part of the

S&D game but to do so would be unquestionably unethical and unforgivable. So don't go there. Use your power wisely using your feminine charms so that he does not want to resist anything you suggest.

PART FOUR: PERFORM THE ACT

The Process

In this section, we will have various scenarios described in the male sub subspace of BDSM. The scenarios should be able to help you plan your own scenes and get you started on the journey to male submission. It will use examples of scenes that can be acted out or simply expanded upon using your imagination. We'll examine various kinds of relationships in which scenes can occur and how they come about and how they take place.

Mounting

Not all d/s relationships are formalized by use of a contract or agreed upon scenes. It can start because a submissive male tries to pin a casual female acquaintance's arms above her head in bed. This could lead to her wrenching her wrists free, shoving him off and leaving him blinking but well-mannered, not touching her. He might not realize that just because she throws him around doesn't mean she wants him to throw her around.

It's different when it's the other way, and that's true for both of them.

She might discover that the male sub craves touch in a way that other guys do not. He wants to be petted and stroked, feel her fingers tighten in his hair and around his arms, five points of pressure digging into his skin. He arches into her as she coasts her palms down his chest. If she pulls back just to test him, he scrambles to fill the empty space, to press tight against the heat of her skin again. He makes desperate sounds when she puts him where she wants them: drags his hands over her own hips, presses his fingers between her legs, and brings his knuckles to her mouth to kiss.

And if she doesn't put his arms above his head, he'll do it for her, and then wait for her fingers to find his wrists like cuffs. She might be able to hold him without effort, and he likes that he can't break her grip no matter how hard he seems to try. The femdom likes that too.

The male sub might be hesitant for a while, compliant. He doesn't make a move without her telling him to make it first. She will sit on the edge of her bed still dressed from jacket to boots and make him take his clothes off, get on his knees, and lick her until she comes or she might sit on his face. Alternatively, she could hold him down and ride him until those barriers he builds up brick by brick are gone and he's shivering, his eyes closed and skin flushed, writhing and not moving even when she takes her hands off him. Staying where she put him. Falling apart. And all the while she gets to remain composed. In control.

When they're done his hair is darkened with sweat and

his face relaxed. Then the femdom gathers him up in her arms and tucks his hair behind his ear. Then she can allow herself to be tender and to be vulnerable.

Arousal and Denial

This scene works well when a male sub goes to see a pro domme, possibly not for the first time. The domme studies the scene before her. He is on his knees, begging without saying words. He is wearing panties and nothing else, his cock forming an obvious bulge in the silk thong. She sits in front of him, in her underwear, dark navy lacy lingerie, legs spread just enough. "So what should I do with you?" She asks leaning forward watching his eyes shift from her face to cleavage, then between her legs before meeting her eyes again.

"Anything Mistress wants…"

"Anything?"

He nods and the mistress stands, her heels causing her to tower over him more a lot more than normal.

"Do you want to be a little slut?" she steps closer, bringing his head level with her wet pussy; the only thing separating him from it is a few inches and a thin strip of fabric. He looks down again and this time she acts on his roaming eyes. "Did I say you could look at my pussy?"

"No mistress,"

"Then why are you?"

"Because... I uh..."

"Answer   me.   Now."
"N-no!"

The mistress smiles, knowing what he is begging for.

"You want to eat my pussy baby?" she asks sweetly cupping his chin so he can look directly at her.

"Yes please, mistress,"

"I've got something better for you, my good little whore." She says.

Moments later she is equipped with a strap-on, the large faux cock inches from his face. "Open your mouth."

Lips sealed, he shakes his head no; she presses the tip to his lips and sternly speaks,

"Open."

His lips part hesitantly and she pushes the dick into his mouth, her hand on the back of his head, guiding him as he bobs his head.

"Good boy," She smiles down at him, locking eyes so she can see his expression as she forces the entire cock down his throat and begins to move slowly, fucking his throat. He pulls away, gagging causing her to smile.

"Did he like that baby? Being Mistress' good little cock whore?"

"Mmm!"

"Say it."

"I like it!"

"Say 'I'm Mistress' cock whore'" She commands holding the cock, wet with his saliva, aimed at his face.

"Go on."

"I'm Mistress' cock whore..." He practically moans, his hand reaching down to rub his aching erection through his thong.

"Don't you dare touch your cock without my permission slut!" she would hiss, glaring at him, his hand had just met his dick and he is reluctant to extract it.

"You know what happens if you touch yourself without my permission."

"I get punished..."

He massages it gently.

"Hands behind your back. Now," she says as she walks across the room to grab the handcuffs from a drawer, purposely bending over to show her thong off to its full extent, knowing he is watching. After she handcuffs him securely, she sits back down, leaving him cuffed and on his knees. She can see how swollen his cock had gotten, the cock ring not helping anything. She takes off the strap-on and begins to rub the tip of the fake cock along his panties. "You are to watch me fuck myself and you will do nothing to please yourself after I come you are to suck the dick clean of my juices and then bend over like a good fuck toy so I can use your ass. Is that clear?"

"Yes Mistress," He glances down, cheeks pink.

She slides her panties off slowly, watching him watching her. She rubs the tip of the fake cock against her slit, parting her wet pussy lips. She teases her clit before pushing the cock into herself slowly. He stares, desperately as she begins moving the dildo quickly in and out while moaning as the pleasure coils in her core. He whimpers and her moaning grows louder as pleasure pulses between her legs.

Her eyes stay on him as she asks, "You like that little slut? Watching mistress fuck herself?" Her words are separated by moans as she begins to reach her climax, her cunt gripping the cock making it go harder, and faster.

He can barely speak as he nods eyes desperate and hungry as she peaks, coming. She slowly pulls out the cock and puts it back on, the plastic shiny with her white liquids. "Come to me. Remain on your knees." He obeys. "Suck it clean." He does, taking the come-soaked cock in its entirety, bobbing his head without her hand guiding him.

"Good little cock whore, sucking Mistress' come off the cock like a good slut." she pulls the cock out of his mouth and tells him that it is enough, he did a good job. She stands up, telling him to do so as well.

 "Lean over on the bed, keep your feet on the ground." she stands behind him, undoing the handcuffs before she positions herself. She pushes it into him slowly, smirking as he groans, gripping the sheets.

"Beg."

"Please Mistress, fuck my ass."

"C'mon you can do better than that, I know how big of a slut you are, beg for Mistress' cock." "Mistress', please fuck my ass! Please, I'm a cock whore please!"

"Good boy..." She thrusts deeply into him and then out before steadying herself to a nice pace. He grabs the sheets, moaning and whining. She smirks, moving faster.

"Do you still want to play with your cock?"

"Mmm!"

"Play with your cock while Mistress' fucks your ass. Don't you dare come!"

"Thank you!" One hand disappears the vibrator on the

strap-on buzzing against her clit slowly drawing her to climax.

It's not long before he's begging to come, but she denies him.

"You may not come until Mistress is finished using you, is that clear?"

"But Mistress!"

She thrusts even harder, "Excuse me?"

"Yes, Mistress."

"That's what I thought." she moans, nearing her second orgasm, watching him moan underneath her causing her to moan even louder. She comes hard as he moans her name again. Slowly, she pulls out of him.

"Good boy, taking Mistress's cock like a good slut!" she praises, taking off the dildo.

"I think you earned a reward."

"Really Mistress?" His eyes go wide and excited, practically bouncing at the thought.

"Really baby, now come here," she says patting beside her.

He scooted closer, and she kisses him, her hand moving down to his throbbing erection, removing the cock ring. He moans in relief as she firmly grasps his swollen cock. Still lip locked, she begins to gently massage him, and she feels him tense up as the pleasure builds. Moving faster she pulls away from the kiss only slightly, his tongue still hungrily looking for hers.

"He like that baby?" she whispers, feeling him throb in her hand.

"Y-yes Mistress!"

"Come for me!"

Come shoots from his cock, covering her hand and she smiles at him, licking it from her fingers. "You're such a good boy."

Cuckoldry and Emasculation

The cuckolding subculture is a subspace of the sexually dominant role where the male sub is known as the cuckold. Cuckolding does not only involve sexual intercourse with another man while the male sub watches. It can range from vocalizing fantasies about other men within a monogamous relationship. For example, "Oh my God, Brad Pitt is so hot. I would let him eat me out so hard."

The more extreme end of cuckolding involves an alternative lifestyle where the cuckoldress selects lovers from outside her primary relationship while the cuckold is expected to remain loyal to her, meet all her needs and accept the humiliation of his position without complaint. The male sub revels in the humiliation and so does the cuckoldress.

The male sub may be restricted from participating in any kind of sexual intercourse up to and including masturbating himself unless specifically allowed by the cuckoldress. She may choose to enforce this by making him wear a chastity belt and keeping the keys on her person at all times. Meanwhile, she chooses other men, known as bulls, to play with. She might have long-term bulls or short-term ones or keep one or two on rotation as she wishes and at her discretion. The sub is forced to deal with the humiliation and emasculation including sometimes watching or participating in her sexual escapades to further his humiliation. She can go so far as to make him have sex with one of her bulls.

Like most d/s relationships, the couple usually signs a contract, which lays out the terms of their relationship. As in any d/s, the domme had power and control over their lives both romantic and non-romantic. This includes having power over their finances.

"I cannot be dominant in this relationship and have sexual power and domination over you without being in control of everything else." She would say, "This is how we make it real."

In addition to financial control, some cuckoldresses prefer that their subs are also house hubbies and they tend to all the household chores. They have dinner waiting when she gets home from work, kiss her on the cheek and ask her how her day was. They take off her shoes and bring her slippers and a drink and sit her down to give her a massage to soothe her tired muscles. He might do this even on occasions where she gets home from a session with one of her bulls.

Should the sub fail in his duties, then he is subject to punishment in any way that she desires. She might take a hairbrush to spank him with, handcuff him to the radiator and leave him there, naked, overnight, suspend him from a hanging contraption or have him wear his chastity belt or a cock ring for long periods of time.

Sometimes the sub not only watches his domme with other men, he is the one who finds these other men for her. These conditions are pre-negotiated before the relationship begins and if the sub is strongly opposed to a certain thing, he can put his foot down and say no and have it included in the contract. Failure to adhere to these contractual agreements puts the relationship at risk.

Even though it's not mandatory for all cuckolds to be married to their partner they need to have a certain level of commitment so as to heighten the erotic high induced from the sexual double standard. You can't be cuckolded if you don't care or are not invested in the other party. This subculture is also associated with exhibitionism and voyeurism since key elements of the scene include putting herself on display while he watches.

Cuckolding tends to begin when a couple are swingers rather than strictly from the BDSM lifestyle. It is a gateway into female sexual dominance. The cuckoldress is separated from the dominatrix in that with the latter, it may be mostly a professional occupation even though some do take it into their personal lives while for the former it's an everyday lifestyle in every way. The cuckoldress plays the role of domme in her primary relationship while the dominatrix satisfies the kink mostly as part of a scene.

The cuckoldress looks for bulls with a larger penis than that of her primary partner and this also adds to his humiliation since it is like he is the loser in a fight to 'win' over their mate using his physical attributes. The difference here is that the sub revels in the humiliation because they are masochistic. In this subspace, all the sub's feelings are intensified. And their mind and emotions are immersed in the present moment. This space has no room for burdens or worries or responsibilities. He is free of the need to make decisions or think. All he has to do is obey.

For those of who don't necessarily equate sex with love, cuckolding should present no emotional risks and it should be easy to switch on and off and treat the experience as the fun escapade it is intended to be. However, it is immensely important for both parties of the committed couple to be completely transparent about their feelings in connection with cuckolding. This is when a contract becomes important. If the man is hurt by seeing his woman having sex with another man, then the practice should be halted immediately. He might have not been sure when he suggested it or agreed to it that was going to be his reaction until he tested it. Emotional literacy can be a flexible attribute that does not always present in a predictable manner. It can also make a difference when the bull is a person who is not trusted or liked by the sub. Although the aim is ultimately to undermine him, and subjugate his masculinity, the level of doing so is a fine line and can potentially result in breakdown of the relationship, especially if the domme becomes emotionally attached to the bull too. It is therefore important to confer with both the domme and the sub about each individual bull; otherwise the experience could be diminished and negate any excitement of the process of cuckolding.

The sub might be excluded from watching the domme and the bull during the actual experience, but it could be filmed so that he is made to watch later. Alternatively, the domme might watch it later whilst making the sub lick her pussy. If the bull is a dom and she acts as a sub with him, and then reverts back to norm with her own partner, this can be perceived as being lower in the pecking order by the couple. She can also make it clear that he must exist purely to ensure she is fully serviced and bring home a different partner of his choice each week or month. However, be careful not to be too random in the choice. Don't for example pick up some undesirable who might not be as hygienic as you would desire. Lay down guidelines to set out quite carefully what you will accept and what is absolutely not acceptable. And remember to agree between you a safety word, which either can use so that the other knows what action should be taken and under what circumstances. Always have the facility to enable you to summon help, even if that does mean calling 911 and getting the police to the rescue.

Punishment

This will be illustrated by playing out a scenario in order to cover a few kinks as well as jumpstart your imagination on ways to carry out punishment.

A couple pulls into a mall's parking lot and she parks the car. This excursion will not be a normal one as he sits in the passenger's seat, looking slightly uncomfortable. The reason for that is the fact he has a cock ring on, a thong, along with a large butt plug - all of that concealed under his pants. She steps from the car, a smirk playing on her face as her heeled boots click against the concrete.

"C'mon," she says.

Her attire is less than modest, pumps, a tight skirt and lots of cleavage. Today she dressed with a cause. She grabs her purse, which contains more surprises.

They enter the large building, going from store to store browsing. She is purposefully going slowly, as he shifts from foot to foot. The plug has been in for almost an hour and a half, along with the ring. She knows his dick is getting swollen and starting to ache. They go to

Victoria's Secret, picking out some new underwear for the both of them. He looks immensely horny, needy and agitated. A few more stores and she decides a dressing room with no employees lurking will be the perfect place to perform his punishment.

She leads him into a large dressing room and pulls the curtain closed. She turns around and sternly says, "Strip down to your panties."

"Yes, Mistress." His face is reddening as she puts her purse on one of the hooks and sits down on the plastic chair in the corner in front of the full-length mirror that covers the wall. "On your knees,"

He obeys, looking down as she decides what to do first. "Crawl to me." She unzips her skirt, pulling it down revealing her black lacy thong. Spreading her legs wide she grabs him by the back of the head, pressing his face against her cunt, and grinding herself against him.

"Do you know why you're being punished?"

He speaks, his words vibrating against her cunt. She feels herself getting wetter and wetter.

"You emptied yourself into me." she says in disgust, "Filling me with your come without permission. You didn't have permission to come either. And when I told you to stop you kept fucking me. You broke lots of rules you little slut."

He nods his head.

"Now I'm going to play with you until I think you've fulfilled your punishment. It's not over until I say and I'd be wary of breaking any more rules."

He nods again because he knows better than to start to eat her before she gives him permission.

"Give it a kiss baby," she commands and he does so, his lips going wet with her juices. She reaches up and pulls on a large, thick dildo and a strap. His eyes go wide as she presses the dildo between her pussy's lips. "Kiss it baby, but don't touch my cunt."

He nods, kissing the dildo while her juices drip down it. She twists the base and it begins to vibrate, buzzing against her clit causing her to moan lightly.

She slips it into herself, "Keep kissing it and be mindful not to touch my cunt."

She fucks herself until come coats the dildo and his mouth. "Clean my hole and the dildo."

He licks it all up.

"Good boy."

She studies him, his cock thick with veins. She could tell it is in need of relief, but she feels like toying with him a bit longer. "I'm sorry, I'm being rude. You need some pleasure too. Stand up, bend over,"

He does as he is told and she places her hands on his hips, moving down to his ass. He whimpers as she slowly pulls out the butt plug. She walks around to his face, "Open. Now."

He shakes his head in refusal but, she grabs his face, "I'm not asking again."

He opens his mouth, casting his eyes away pouting.

"Good boy."

She returns to his ass, teasing him a little more before sliding two fingers inside of him, loosening him for the large faux dick about to rip him apart.

"You like that little slut?"

"Mmm, yes mistress,"

"You want a cock in your ass, whore?"

"Please..."

She attaches the dildo to the strap and puts it on rubbing it against his entrance before slowly pushing it in. He moans quietly, small cries slipping from his mouth.

"Shh baby, we can't have anyone hear us," She slams the entire length roughly into him and he cries out. She pounds his ass as he fists his hands, knuckles turning white as desperate sounds slip from his mouth.

"May I please touch my cock?" He begs, whimpering every syllable.

"This is a punishment ass slut; don't think I'm going to let you receive any pleasure."

"Y-yes ma'am." he lifts his ass higher, his upper body pushing down, head bowed.

"Good slut."

She fucks his ass until she is satisfied, coming against the vibrator on the strap-on twice to his desperate, pathetic moans. She slowly pulls out, leaving him gasping for air, trying to control his breathing.

"Lie down."

He obeys, looking up at her; she slowly lowers her ass onto his face suffocating him.

"Begin eating me."

His tongue hungrily licks away, moaning into her. "You may touch yourself, whore." He thanks her, muffled as he moans louder, she watches him please his swollen cock, hand moving quickly over his large vein covered member.

He begins begging to come, the vibrations of his voice against her ass and pussy caused her to get even hornier.

She stands and says, "Come on your face. Now."

"Thank you, Mistress!!" He moans closing his eyes in relief as a hot load shoots from his cock splattering against his cheeks and mouth.

She runs her finger along his face, scooping up the come. "Look at this mess," she offers her finger to his mouth and he graciously sucks it clean, swirling his tongue around her finger.

"Good boy," she pulls her finger from his mouth, whipping more come from his face, then bringing the same finger to her mouth, locking eyes with him as she licks it clean.

She redresses herself and then dresses him, whipping off the dildo before putting it and the butt plug away, along with his cock ring. She kisses him gently, dripping with passion and love.

"I love you, baby,"

He smiles against her lips, "I love you too,"

And with that, they leave the mall hand in hand.

Of course, this is the perfect scenario and the dimension of being caught adds to the thrill. Don't put yourself at risk though of being arrested for lewd behavior and appearing on the national news. Whilst it might be stimulating to imagine that you could be caught, the reality of it could be very different and mar one or both of you for life. You should also be used to your partner's pain threshold and have tested your own strength on him previously. Fucking him with a dildo is fine providing you know what you're doing but be careful of not submitting him to physical internal damage. Caution is best so play it safe and interpret tough love with care.

Pet Play

She pats his head and he purrs, low in his chest, as she walks around him. She pulls her hand back and taps his chin so his blindfolded face will look up and kisses him, softly. Once she's done, he mumbles. "Thank you, mistress."

"Good boy." She coos, pushing his head back down. Then she keeps pushing until he's back on all fours.

He's sweating a bit, and she tugs his reins forward until he starts a slow canter around her. He wickers like a horse quietly, and whinnies when she stops him. After trailing her hand down his spine, she tugs, just barely, on the tailed plug in his waste chute. He whimpers, his bulge lashing slightly.

"Do you think you've been a good pony?" She asks, petting his smooth hair. He purrs, his shoulders going slack. Well, that just won't do. Quick as a snake, she brings the crop down on one round of his buttocks and he snaps to attention.

"I think you need to be punished."

He whinnies again and stays almost completely still as she guides his bulge into his nook, only making the barest of whines as it stretches him. She trails the tip of the crop along his spine and he shivers trembles even as his bulge lashes around inside him. Her own bulge is twisting against her thigh under her skirt, and she wants nothing more than to push his face into the floor and take him from behind, but his nook is currently being used for his cute little display of self-torture.

But then, it's not as if she can't use something else. She kneels behind him and shoves his shoulders down, luckily not having to strain against his real strength. Once he's in that perfectly submissive position, she crouches over him and bites the back of his neck, slowly twisting the smallish, bulb-shaped toy out of him. He whimpers and his claws scrabble at the ground, a thin string of drool trailing from his lips as his mouth opens in a smooth moan. She watches his eyes roll back as she finally removes the plug with a soft pop.

Then, she lifts her skirt daintily and presses her bulge in, her breath catching in her throat for a moment. That feels *good*. He mewls softly and rocks his hips back to meet her shallow thrusts, face flickering between enjoying it and hating it. Soon, though, he's gone, lost in the strange pleasure as she tells him how he feels.

"You're so good. You take my bulge so well. Don't you like my bulge?" She licks the slightly pointed ear by her face and he shudders.

"I... I l-love your bulge."

She brings the crop down on his shoulder blade.

"Pardon?"

"I love your bulge... Mistress... Ahn..." His thighs are starting to tense, and she speeds her pace a bit.

In only a little while, she comes, filling him with material and watching his pretty, sweat-stained face twist as she does. When she pulls her withering bulge out of him, he shivers. After only a half-second of thought, she pops the tail back into him, effectively keeping him from spilling anything. He looks at her pleadingly.

"It feels strange, mistress." He licks his lips. "Not, Uhm." He pauses as she presses on the exposed area of his bulge, hips snapping into the contact and body nearly-only nearly-going lax. "Not bad strange, though, mistress, but lewd."

She nips the sensitive point of his ear and he whimpers. "You like being my bucket then?"

He nods, his sticky hair shaking.

"Out loud." She leaves a lovely cobalt mark on his ass with her crop.

"Y-yes, I love being your bucket, mistress. Thank you, mistress."

"Do you want to come for me?"

"Yes, please, mistress." He mumbles, biting his bottom lip as she presses at his bulge.

"Only if you don't spill a drop." She coos, working two, then three fingers into him and rubbing against the front wall of his nook.

He shouts a yes, rolling his hips and moving as well as he can, thighs trembling. She sucks little marks on his skin, in the dips on either side of his spine as she works her fingers in him. His bulge is flicking inside him hard, and his breathing is ragged and hot. She can't help but notice the slight pool of drool on the floor next to his face, and the translucent blue lubricant running down his thighs.

Soon enough, he's pushing himself up, making little whines and high-pitched noises she has come to know signal his release. When he looks back at her, lips trying and failing to form the wordless moans spilling from them into proper syntax, she kisses his shoulder.

"Come for me."

And he does, filling his own nook and making a warble that makes her want to fuck him again. He pants, arms shivering, as his bulge and her fingers slip out of his nook and he tries not to spill any. She moves to his front and pepper little kisses on his face, stroking his hair and telling him how well he did. Then, she whispers in his ear.

"Do you need to stop?"

He shakes his head, breathing still harsh. "Please, no."

She kisses him, full on the lips, and he says thank you.

Body Worship

The male sub's cock slid into the Domme's wet inviting pussy and she smiled wickedly because his rigid member felt so good inside her. The view of his ass in the strategically placed mirror heightened the feeling. He stood slightly stooped at the edge of the bed thrusting slowly in and out of her.

He did not have permission to go any faster just yet. She enjoyed watching the redness of his ass and the delightful cane welts across his upper thighs as he labored on her behalf. Her male sub was such a brave boy taking the pain for her pleasure.

She absolutely relished punishing him when he displeased her, but sometimes she just wanted to cane, whip or spank him just for fun. With her considerable skill and experience, she could easily make him feel the difference between a punishment and foreplay.

"Hold it inside," she commanded.

He obeyed, burying himself to the hilt and staying pressed against her until she said otherwise. She gripped his ass and laughed as she saw him wince.

"Okay. You may speed up. But just a little! And don't

you dare come yet."

He followed her instructions to the letter, staying in control even as he raised the tempo of his thrusts. His eyes went to the other implements she wouldn't hesitate to use on his still tender flesh if he were to disobey. She wouldn't contain his punishment to just his backside. His balls would also pay for his misdeeds. So it was better to wait for her permission before losing himself completely. Unless he was feeling particularly frisky.

"Stop," she ordered.

He withdrew immediately, taking a step back. There was a worried expression on his face. She let him wonder what was coming for a moment, knowing he was waiting to see if he was in trouble or if perhaps she was going to leave him unsatisfied all night. He looked like he was about to ask for permission to speak but she preempted him.

"We will change positions."

She curled up and rolled over. Scooting back over in front of him, she bent forward and raised her ass up in front of him. Spreading her legs, she braced herself with her forearms.

"I want you to go deeper. Same speed, no coming yet."

He nodded his acquiescence and hastened to do as she said.

Stepping forward and pulling his cock down into position, he slid back inside her. They both gasped. He worked his way back into the rhythm she had commanded.

"Oh, Mistress. Oh, Mistress! I love your pussy!"

"I did not tell you, you could speak!" she spat before moaning, arching her back and coming. It was her third time that night.

Then she rested on her arms, making him await her verdict for his disobedience as he trembled inside her.

"Does my slave want to come?"

"Yes please, Mistress!" he said. "Please?"

"Hmm," she teased. "You may speed up and come."

He sped up. She could feel every muscle inside him tensing as he got right to the edge. She could feel the mix of desire and frustration flowing through him as he couldn't seem to get himself over that edge and into the orgasmic bliss he so desired. That bliss she knew she owned that he had surrendered totally to her. She helped him along by saying, "Come for me, slave!"

He exploded inside her. A loud low moan issued from his lips as his semen filled the condom wrapped around his cock. Several smaller moans followed as his cock continued spurting. He slowed his thrusts, and then stopped altogether. Sliding out of her pussy, he half-collapsed onto the bed. Breathing heavily, he could barely make out his next words between gasps. Still, he managed to say, "Thank you, Mistress."

After disposing of the condom, they cuddled. He was still breathing heavily and trembling as they held each other.

Taking it Step-by-Step

This may all sound like pretty advanced behavior, especially if you're new to it. The trick is to take things very slowly, only rarely do two people get together for a BDSM experience and manage to shake off their inhibitions immediately, simultaneously and completely. If you decide to draw up a contract, don't just write it up and forget it. Refer to it regularly, which is not to say immediately before each session. You don't want to lose any spontaneity you may have felt but bear in mind what you last agreed, which may well change over time. Don't ever criticize openly what your partner tries. You are bound to make mistakes as you feel your way and things, which you expected to like and turn out to disgust you or completely turn you off, might surprise you. Try your best to be open about what you want. If your partner does something you don't like, tell him, but do so constructively, not super-critically. This can be a fine line to tread bearing in mind that the S&D relationship is one of dominance. But it doesn't have to brutally and indefinitely denigrate his self-confidence, it's more about carefully leading him to where you want him to be.

Being aware of each other's feelings and sensibilities can be an indication of how deeply you love and trust each other. This doesn't give either of you license to hurt the other or go against their wishes. Agree what is acceptable to you as a couple because it is about mutual satisfaction. Both of you should gain by the experience. When an imbalance occurs, and there is no mutual satisfaction, the experience can become destructive and force the couple apart.

When I used to adopt the submissive role, I often kept quiet about things I didn't want to happen because I thought it was pleasing my partner. I put up with pain that I did not welcome, and which did nothing to excite me sexually. This situation continued for a protracted amount of time until one day he overstepped the boundary of my pain threshold completely and we ended up having a huge row. It turned out that he had got no pleasure from hurting me either but was performing in such a way because he thought that's what I wanted. I cannot stress strongly enough that communication lines should always be open and if there is anything at all that you are not happy with, speak up. Try not to leave it until the actual act is taking place because whatever speech occurs in the height of passion might easily be misconstrued as being part of the sex play.

Getting to know your partner is a gradual process and that's why it must be taken step by step. If it's something that you want to introduce into your sex lives, then try not to rush as it like a bull at a gate. Be patient with your partner. He might be doing his very best to please you and give you what you want but he is likely to feel self-conscious as well at first so talk about it in detail before you get down to the brass tacks of it.

If it's something that you are introducing into your sex lives for the first time, try to introduce the topic at an opportune time when he is relaxed and in the right environment. Driving to the supermarket when he's trying to escape rush hour traffic would not be a good time for instance. It might be a good idea to dress up a little wearing appropriate clothing to give him the idea. You don't necessarily have to invest huge sums in rubber and leather garments or lots of sex toys. Be inventive. Sex is creative and this is where you can show your creativity at its best.

It might be a good idea to set the scene and surprise him when he gets home from work. Dress in your sexiest gear and have a meal that you can share waiting for him. Ply him with soft music and alcohol. You could initiate things by undoing his pants and then revealing that you are not wearing any underwear before mounting him where he sits. You could then progress onto bending over the dining table in front of him and telling him to lick your pussy dry. The evening could then progress by leading him to the bedroom and telling him to undress you. If you don't normally shave your pubes, surprise him that day. Wear high heels and stockings and tell him to stop when that is all you are wearing. Then command him to undress completely and lie flat on the bed. You could sit on his face before typing his hands down and mounting him again. First steps should be tentative. There is little doubt that he will be turned on by your actions, which don't have to include whipping or pain, at least not at first. He should respond in much the same way a dog does, responding to praise and treats. Only ever inflict pain after he has consented to it and said that he wants that to be part of your sex life together.

There is no wrong or right; if you are both happy with what is occurring then it is okay and should be continued. Review what went before after every session and be honest if you want to have more or less of what has occurred. Allow your partner to do the same and actively listen to what he says and act upon it. To proceed with actions regardless of his feelings is a dangerous way to go and you put the relationship in jeopardy. S&D relationships only work well because of the high level of trust you must put in another person. If that is destroyed or ignored, then you run the risk of the relationship disintegrating.

Making Mistakes

It's almost inevitable that one or both of you will make mistakes along the way. It would be highly unusual for everything to work out perfectly on the first session or indeed on every session. The most valuable thing you can take away from a mistake is to learn from it and be open to constructive criticism. Welcome it as a chance to learn and don't take gently criticism personally.

Encourage your partner to say what he has enjoyed and what he disliked. Communication is a two-way mechanism and channels should always be open, even if not actively encouraged during the actual session. It's a joint learning opportunity and a chance for you to both grow sexually and emotionally too, barring those times when one of you needs to use the safe word, of course.

It's easy to go too far in the heights of passion or because you misunderstand his reaction. Perhaps you hurt him too much physically or upset him by touching a nerve, which you were unaware, was an issue with him. Encourage him to say so. If he stays quiet in the mistaken belief that he thinks that is what you want of him, resentment will begin to grow, and the longer things are left unsaid the easier it is for things to fester and destroy your relationship. If you detect that he might be sulking after a session for instance, then use that as an opportunity to get him to open up to you. He's already agreed that he trusts you to abuse him physically but intimacy on this level also leads to an emotional intimacy where your partner should feel freer to discuss issues, which he might never have shared with anyone else. This is a way to connect on the deepest level possible so don't just try and brush mistakes under the carpet thinking they will go away. They won't and if you keep on making the same mistake repeatedly you are ignoring an excellent opportunity of moving your relationship to a deeper level.

Don't take yourselves too seriously. Sex should be fun, no matter how you choose to find gratification. For instance, if your body inadvertently makes embarrassing noises, then laugh at yourself. Undue seriousness can come over as sinister and scary. Try not to be too intense. If you are too grim and sober sex can feel seedy rather than sexy.

Talk about your past mistakes with your partner to put him at ease and help to rid him of his inhibitions. If either of you feel silly or foolish it is going to prove difficult for you to enjoy a relaxed but passionate session. Instead of laughing at each other, learn to laugh together at the mistakes that either or your make. To balance out any gentle criticism, interject it with positive words and praise about what he did do right. Obviously, you might be telling him what a bad boy he is but make it plain that this is all part of the game and doesn't diminish your affection for him.

The better you get to know your partner, the easier reading his signals becomes but new relationships always present different challenges. Don't ever assume that one person will like the same things as your last partner. We are all different. That's why it's so important to start off gently. If you start trying to introduce the heavy stuff straightaway, you might drive that potential hot lover away quicker than you had hoped. By the same token, it's just as big a mistake to stay silent about your own sexual preferences. I'm not suggesting that you tell him on your first date but as your relationship develops, he might even ask you what you like sexually. This is your time to speak up and tell him. If he does run a mile, quietly muttering that you're a freak, was it ever going to work anyway? Let it go. Whilst some people might say that sex is not everything, it is a pretty important element in a relationship and at its best can bond a couple together and get them over a lot of hurdles. If you are aware that S&D is always going to be a fundamental facet of your sex life, then do say so before the relationship goes too far though and you are both invested in it emotionally. Having that one thing drive you apart can be just as painful if it is not possible to decide on a compromise and find a central path through.

Don't make the mistake that all men will be the same and appreciate being dominated, however sexy and appealing the woman is. Some males will be deeply entrenched in their masculinity and enjoy being dominant themselves, unwilling to ever enjoy being submissive. If it's someone you have high hopes in, then it's a shame and up to you to decide if it's possible for you to deny your true feelings. But be honest with yourself and your potential partner because it's not fair to them either if you pretend to be someone you're not. Can you really imagine the rest of your sex life being unfulfilled and unsatisfying? It's up to you to decide your priorities. Do it sooner rather than later. It is far preferable than going behind their backs and seeking sexual fulfillment with someone else. The level of intimacy possible in an honest and caring relationship is worth the wait until you find the right person so that you can take each other to heights that you might never do with the wrong person trying his hardest to be the right one.

After A Session

This is the time for tenderness, a time for holding each other, cuddling and declaring your everlasting love for the other person. Stroke each other and kiss gently in non-erogenous areas. It's a cooling off period and an opportunity to reassure the other person that it has brought you much closer together because you shared total trust between you. Say that you appreciate having such a loving relationship.

Participating in an S&D session is likely to be very powerful and can dredge up all sorts of feelings and emotions, sometimes ones that are difficult to filter or decipher. It might even be that your partner remembers something in detail that he had managed to file away, and he gets extremely upset. You have to know how you're going to deal with this because it is likely that you will feel responsible and he may feel he is struggling how to cope and where to go from there. Don't let this spoil any future sessions. Nip it in the bud and deal with it and if he needs help to put himself together again, do it together and be there to support him. It's important that after every session the couple discuss what happened. This is especially true if the partnership is a long-term, stable one. Each partner must feel happy about what happened and feel free to say so if they did not. Discuss which aspects of the session you particularly liked and try to say why. Ask your partner to do the same. Not only can this help to bond you even closer, it can also prolong the erotica. It's not healthy to keep doubts inside of you because if left to fester a small problem can easily elevate to what seems an insurmountable obstacle that can potentially ruin any sexual inclination. Neither of you should continue to take part in an action just to please the other person because this evolves into an unequal union. If one partner was unhappy with an aspect of the session, agree between you that it should not be used again or at least find ways in which you could adapt it so that it is acceptable. It's about negotiation and compromise, but that's what loving another person involves and comes as part of the package. It's the whole deal.

Considering how physically intimate you have been with your partner, talking about something intimate you did should not present a problem. To have this type of relationship at all requires you to have total confidence in another person and to place your entire trust in them to look after you and have those feelings reciprocated. If either of you do not feel this way then perhaps it is too soon for you to set off down this road. At the very least you need to discuss how and where you start. Every one of us will be at a different stage in their sexual development and desire to expand it.

Of course, it is natural that you are going to feel nervous and have a mixture of emotions that you might never have experienced previously. Try to divorce these feelings of excitement and anticipation from any feelings of foreboding. If you or your partner still feels an aversion to S&D, you need more discussion, or perhaps it is not for you at all. And should either of you definitely not want to pursue an S&D relationship, the other partner should not put any pressure on them to do so because the relationship becomes unequal. There should be no emotional blackmail involved because this could seriously put your relationship at risk. Hopefully, after much discussion and experimentation you will be able to find a way through with your partner to enjoy a satisfying S&D partnership.

If it is just one or a couple of aspects of the session that you or your partner are unhappy about, try and talk through why the other person feels like they did. Sex is a powerful tool of the kit we all possess and is one that we should all enjoy to its fullest potential. But everyone has different motivations and sexual triggers so under no circumstances make the other person feel inadequate. Just because you are using the medium of S&D for enjoyment does not mean that you should not cherish him and respect his feelings at all times.

If it does bring up something from the past that has been locked away because it caused too much pain, then seek help from a professional counselor. Each of us is an extremely complex, living being and we must learn to accept that sex is for enjoyment, not just procreation. But with the right partner, sex can be a miraculous gift, which is there for us all to explore and experiment with. As long as it is performed between two consenting adults, then whatever rocks your boat should be enjoyed in all its glory. If you find someone with whom you are simpatico and who enjoys the same things as you do sexually hang onto them. You might not be quite there yet, but it can be enormous fun on the journey as well as arriving. Enjoy yourselves!

Conclusion

There is not much data out there on male submission possibly due to the sensitive nature of the subject. Hopefully, this book gives enough of a roadmap to let you know what you're getting into.

Before You Go

Please leave and honest Amazon review and don't forget to visit my site alexandramorris.com

Check out my other books:

Erotic Hypnosis

Kink 101
Introduction to the submissive lifestyle

References

https://submissiveguide.com/dsrelationships/articles/are-female-dominants-more-about-mental-dominance-than-physical-dominance?series=series-for-male-submissives

https://submissiveguide.com/dsrelationships,%20personalgrowth,%20fundamentals/series/series-for-male-submissives

http://www.clubfem.com/ref_contract.htm

https://submissiveguide.com/personalgrowth/articles/male-submission-selfishness/related.1

https://www.scribd.com/document/293953133/An-Owned-Life

https://www.lelo.com/blog/role-call-what-are-different-kinds-dominants-submissives/

https://www.kinkly.com/definition/664/female-dominance-femdom

https://www.revolvy.com/main/index.php?s=Male+submission&item_type=topic

https://greatist.com/play/guide-to-male-female-erogeneous-zones

http://www.rebelcircus.com/blog/men-like-dominated-bed/2/

<http://elisesutton.com/>